# The
# Cancer
## Treatment
## Revolution

# The
# Cancer
## Treatment
## Revolution

## How Smart Drugs and Other New Therapies Are Renewing Our Hope and Changing the Face of Medicine

### David G. Nathan

John Wiley & Sons, Inc.

Published by John Wiley & Sons, Inc., Hoboken, New Jersey
Published simultaneously in Canada

Wiley Bicentennial Logo: Richard J. Pacifico

The information contained in this book is not intended to serve as a replacement for professional medical advice. Any use of the information in this book is at the reader's discretion. The author and the publisher specifically disclaim any and all liability arising directly or indirectly from the use or application of any information contained in this book. A health care professional should be consulted regarding your specific situation.

For general information about our other products and services, please contact our Customer Care Department within the United States at (800) 762-2974, outside the United States at (317) 572-3993 or fax (317) 572-4002.

Wiley also publishes its books in a variety of electronic formats. Some content that appears in print may not be available in electronic books. For more information about Wiley products, visit our web site at www.wiley.com.

*Library of Congress Cataloging-in-Publication Data:*

Nathan, David G., date.
    The cancer treatment revolution : how smart drugs and other new therapies
are renewing our hope and changing the face of medicine / David G. Nathan.
        p.  cm.
    Includes bibliographical references and index.
    ISBN 978-0-471-94654-0 (cloth)
    1. Cancer—Patients.  2. Cancer—Treatment—Popular works.  I. Title.
    RC263.N38  2007
    616.99′4—dc22

                                                        2006024621

Printed in the United States of America

10  9  8  7  6  5  4  3  2  1

*To Jean and the wonderful*
*family she gave me*

# Contents

Ken's Story

# Acknowledgments

I am in debt to the many supporters and colleagues who made this book possible. From the beginning of the project, I received the encouragement, wisdom, and skill of my wonderful agent, Jill Kneerim, and of the president of the Dana-Farber Cancer Institute, Edward J. Benz, Jr., M.D. Initial editing advice came from Steven Marcus. Laura Van Dam became my private editor during the final year of completion of the manuscript. She did a masterful job even while battling her own serious illness. The manuscript was ultimately dissected and improved by Tom Miller, Juliet Grames, and Kimberly Monroe-Hill at Wiley.

The construction of this book required over a score of transcribed interviews with patients and with colleagues who have contributed far more to cancer care and research than I. These and other significant editing expenses were defrayed by generous grants from the Richard and Susan Smith Family Foundation and the Goldhirsh Foundation.

The first draft of the book was assembled during a delightful five-week residence at the Villa Serbelloni of the Rockefeller Foundation in Bellagio, Italy, in the fall of 2003. I am grateful to the foundation and to colleagues who supported my application for the residency. These were Joseph Goldstein, M.D., Phillip Sharp, Ph.D., and Harold Varmus, M.D.

Several colleagues, family members, and friends willingly read sections of this book and gave me excellent critiques. They included Ann Barnet, M.D., the late Richard J. Barnet, Nathaniel I. Berlin, M.D., Sissela and Derek Bok, Thomas Brand, Deborah Charness, George Demetri, M.D., Mimi Dow, Frank H. Gardner, M.D., Judy Holding, Philip Kantoff, M.D., Steven Karp, David Livingston, M.D., Robert Mayer, M.D., Linda Nathan, C. O. North, Ann Partridge, M.D., Orah Platt, M.D., Kornelia Polyak, M.D., Ph.D., Dorothy Puhy, and Jane Weeks, M.D. I have tried to incorporate their suggestions and thank them for their efforts. I am particularly thankful to Samuel J. Cohen for his contributions to the suggested reading list and to David E. Fisher, M.D., and Loren Walensky, M.D., who scanned parts of the manuscript for scientific accuracy. If errors remain, they are mine.

The practical task of assembly of this book fell in order to Janet Cameron, Toby Church, Bernadine B. Kirkland, and Cathy Lantigua. Without their combined effort, the manuscript would still be in tatters.

My wonderful wife, Jean F. Nathan, devoted hour after hour to poring over chapters, forcing rewrites, and asking all the right questions. For this and fifty-five years of helping me in every possible way, I thank her from the bottom of my heart.

Finally, I want to thank the caretakers, cancer researchers, and patients who inspired this book and made it possible. I have vaguely wanted to write about "smart" drugs in cancer for several years. But the story would be as dull as a textbook were it not about real patients and about the physicians, nurses, basic scientists, and support staff who surround them. Mario's family, Joan, and Ken were particularly generous of their time. They did so because they, like the clinicians, nurses, staff members, and researchers, want to help others through the strait gate of cancer. Having suffered, they hope to relieve suffering for others. It is an honor to share their stories and the stories of their caretakers and cancer researchers with my readers.

# Prologue

K en nearly died one night in 1999. He was forty-eight years old and had been treated repeatedly with blood transfusions for unexplained anemia, but never for a minute did he think he was close to death. He was working every day and enjoying life. Then came the night all hell broke loose. He awoke suddenly with terrible abdominal pain and went into shock. If fast-moving EMTs and a savvy surgeon at his community hospital had not realized that Ken required immediate abdominal surgery, he would not have survived the night.

The operation revealed a grapefruit-size tumor attached to his small intestine. Some of the tumor cells had grown into his bowel, leaving a huge hole in his intestine. That night, the contents of Ken's gut had poured into his abdomen and caused terrible inflammation and shock. Worse, the tumor cells had scattered all over his belly. He was doomed to have multiple cancers grow in his abdomen.

A few weeks later, Ken and his wife, Peggy, learned he had a form of cancer that would result in an utterly unmanageable situation when the distributed tumor cells began to grow. He had no traditional treatment options, since the cancer—gastrointestinal stromal tumor, most often called GIST—stubbornly resists radiation and chemotherapy. And its complete surgical removal was impossible. But Peggy did not give up hope. She went on the Internet and found that George Demetri, an oncologist at the Dana-Farber Cancer Institute in Boston, was just a few months away from starting a clinical trial with the first so-called smart drug treatment for tumors like Ken's.

One of the leading physicians interested in GIST, Demetri had learned that a mutation in a single gene in one of the billions of cells in an otherwise healthy body causes the disease. The altered gene, called an oncogene, creates proteins that figuratively shout at cells to divide constantly—that is, to become cancerous. The oncologist also found out that the pharmaceutical company Novartis had developed a drug that should be able to halt the mutated gene's actions by blocking the shouting protein's function, thus killing the cancer. What's more, the drug wasn't supposed to seriously damage any other system in the body. When hundreds of GIST cells that had spread in Ken's abdomen began to grow, Demetri started treating him with the drug. The tumors vanished.

Ken's story illustrates the radically new era on the horizon of cancer therapy—using drugs that are "smart" in that they precisely block the defective genetic pathways that cause and promote cancer. These new compounds destroy cancer cells yet cause minimal damage to normal cells.

The revolution in cancer genetics is giving new hope to everyone, from clinicians and medical researchers to patients and their loved ones. Pharmaceutical companies are quickly developing smart drugs. A few medicines have already passed required testing phases and have entered general oncology clinics for broad use. Within two decades—perhaps even one—a high proportion of cancer patients will receive such treatment. We are already beating back many kinds of aggressive cancers with smart drugs, and we will defeat even more in the years to come.

The global impact of cancer has been bleak. There are approximately fifteen million recorded new cancer cases and at least ten million deaths annually worldwide. There are over one million invasive cancers diagnosed annually in the United States, and more than a half million people die of invasive cancers every year. But survival is at last improving in the United States. As of 2000, there were ten million cancer survivors (including survivors of local cancers) in the United States, for a survival rate of 65 percent. The survivors and the dead represent an economic burden of over $200 billion due to direct medical expenses, morbidity, and concomitant lost productivity.

Cancer research surged after 1971, when President Richard M. Nixon declared the "war on cancer." Almost forty years later, that work has produced some startling victories. With the exception of death from stomach cancers, cancer-related age-specific mortality has recently begun to decline, after a steady rise between the 1930s and the 1990s. Some of the reversal is due to preventive strategies such as campaigns to reduce smoking. Better screening, heightened early detection, and improved combination chemotherapy have also led to much better survival rates.

The medical world has made enormous strides in, for example, childhood cancers (those occurring up through age fourteen). The most common of these, called acute lymphoblastic leukemia, was uniformly fatal until the 1960s. Today, more than 80 percent of the patients with these cancers survive because of treatment with highly toxic but effective combination chemotherapy. Mario's story, the account of a nineteen-month-old boy with a particularly virulent form of childhood leukemia, illustrates that victory. Oncologists have translated many of the pediatric advances and have used combination chemotherapy to help cure adults with certain leukemias and Hodgkin's disease (a cancer of the lymph nodes), breast, testicular, colorectal, and head and neck cancers. The story of Joan, a sixty-two-year-old woman with metastatic breast cancer, describes some of that progress. Improved surgery, radiation therapy, and imaging to delineate cancerous areas have also made important contributions, especially in the management of local cancers.

With smart drugs, even more patients should be able to live for longer periods with far less toxicity. Painting a completely rosy picture about the new compounds isn't fair, however. These drugs have drawbacks that need close attention. The most serious is the development of drug resistance.

*The Cancer Treatment Revolution* will describe the drama and the history of the new era of defeating cancer with smart drugs, using a narrative that focuses on the personal stories of Ken, Mario, and Joan, three patients I knew through my work at the Dana-Farber Cancer Institute and Children's Hospital in Boston. Each of them had a different highly invasive cancer. Their three cases represent the three broad categories of the disease: the sarcomas, the leukemias, and the much more common carcinomas or epithelial cancers. Each of these classes requires a different basic approach to treatment. Medical researchers and pharmaceutical companies are now developing smart drug candidates for all three of these general classes. The stories also form a narrative thread about the development of ever better drugs and techniques to kill cancer. The desperation, creativity, hope, and occasional clashes among the patients and families, doctors and nurses, and cancer researchers are very much part of that long search.

Until recently, Ken's, Mario's, and Joan's cancers were almost certainly lethal. Today, significant hope exists for Mario and Joan, and many patients with Ken's type of widespread sarcoma, which not long ago was considered untreatable, are in complete remission due to smart drugs.

I've been fortunate to have had a first-row seat in observing enormous changes in cancer treatment throughout my career, from serving as a young doctor at the National Cancer Institute in Bethesda, Maryland, to presiding over the Dana-Farber Cancer Institute, and finally working today as a clinician and professor at Harvard Medical School. Readers must understand, however, that my first-row seat, though highly instructive, has not put me in personal contact with the whole world of cancer research. That world is vastly multicentric. Since I have chosen a narrative style to illustrate the advances of the past half century, I have restricted most of my examples to patients and researchers whom I know or knew. But my readers need to appreciate that a universe of important cancer research exists beyond Boston, Massachusetts, and Bethesda, Maryland.

That disclaimer stated, I must say that never before have I felt as confident that oncologists will soon be able to fight many invasive and widespread cancers successfully. I am grateful to Ken and his wife, Peggy, the parents of Mario, and Joan and her family—along with their clinicians and the smart-drug researchers behind the scenes—for letting me share their stories with readers. I have protected the identities of Mario and Joan and their families. Ken wanted his story known in the hope that it will help other cancer victims. The physicians, nurses, and basic scientists at Dana-Farber Cancer Institute and Children's Hospital and those in other institutions who kindly allowed me to interview them have agreed to let me identify them.

When their son was nineteen months old, Mario's parents learned that he had an exceptionally savage form of leukemia. Six years later, he's in remission. His tale will serve both as a review of critical history about fighting cancer with combination (or carpet-bombing) chemotherapy and as an initial look at the possibility of treating cancer with smart drugs based on extensive knowledge about genetic pathways. Only two years before Mario was born, oncologists had come up with the combination chemotherapeutic program that ended up working for him. Now a smart drug that blocks the effects of a gene mutation that contributes to Mario's leukemia is waiting in the wings should he need it in the future.

When she was sixty-two, Joan, a teacher and community service worker, discovered she had breast cancer—one of the most common kinds of cancer—and that her cancer was already in an advanced stage. Breast cancer was the first common tumor that oncologists treated successfully with combination chemotherapy back in the 1970s. Invasive breast cancer—tumors that have spread from the milk ducts to supporting breast tissue and beyond to lymph nodes in the armpit—used to be fatal in 70 percent of patients. Joan's story illustrates how doctors manage the disease today far more effectively with surgery, radiation therapy, and hormone-blocking drugs, as well as with combination chemotherapy. What's more, in 1990, doctors started using the first smart anticancer treatment (not a pill but an antibody given intravenously) to help defeat the kind of cancerous cells found in one of every four breast cancer patients. Taken together, these different forms of treatment now enable nearly 80 percent of patients like Joan to survive and go on to live cancer-free lives.

Ken went through a tremendous amount of medical stress immediately before and after he received a diagnosis of an incurable, fatal cancer. Despite the fact that he was charting new seas of treatment, Ken took one day at a time, eager and grateful for every clinical trial that might offer him more years. He decided early on that his purpose in life was to become a "compass needle" for other patients, telling them they can and should, as needed, seek out cutting-edge smart-drug treatments. "You've got to try to beat the cancer as best you can, with as much dignity as you can," he said.

We have many miles to go on the road of smart-drug development, but the cancer research community has now discovered a path that promises far better tumor treatments in the future. Unfortunately, patients like Mario, Joan, and Ken will risk death before enough smart drugs are developed for them. But the pace of defeating cancer is quickening. This is the time to tell the story about the new method of fighting the disease. Smart drugs are the future of cancer treatment—and the future has started to arrive.

*The Cancer Treatment Revolution* is about three patients with cancer and the scientific progress made over the past fifty years that has entirely changed the future of cancer therapy. Some readers may wish to focus on the stories of the patients. Others may delve into the science, and still others may do both. This book is constructed to allow such freedom of choice, and a bibliography is included for those who want to go to the sources. There is no sin in reading for enjoyment.

# The Nature of the Beast

For as long as we have known about cancer, we have hated and feared it. Cancer is a very inclusive term: there are well over a hundred different subtypes within the three broad classes of invasive cancers, and there are many other cancers (fortunately the vast majority) that tend to remain local. These local cancers are relatively noninvasive and therefore treatable (or curable) by surgery or radiation therapy. People with local cancers now have more than a 90 percent chance of surviving five years if the cancer is surgically removed or destroyed by radiation before it spreads beyond its original site. High rates of recovery can also be achieved with standard combination chemotherapy of many adult cancers even if they have spread to draining lymph nodes and beyond.

Though cancer has been associated with abnormal chromosomes for over a hundred years, the causes of cancer were nearly a complete mystery until the first half of the twentieth century, when genes made of DNA (deoxyribonucleic acid) were shown to control the behavior of cells. Cancer is the result of an abnormal amount or function of specialized proteins that influence cell growth. Therefore, cancer is due to very specific changes or mutations in one or more of our twenty thousand to twenty-five thousand genes, particularly genes that produce proteins that influence the rate and extent of cell division. The genetic damage can arise in any cell of any organ, making cancer the most diverse of any of the major illnesses and the most frequent disease of the human genome.

An invasive cancer (like the cancers described in this book) is an abnormal growth that arises from a single cell and spreads destructively. Like the crab from which it gets its name, invasive cancer moves its claws in all directions, pushing abnormal cells into normal tissue and destroying normal organs in the process. But cancer is as complex as the vital organs in which it arises. Cancer cells are derived from their host organs such as the bone marrow, the breast, and the gastrointestinal tract. Just as these organs are made of many different cell types that create a structure, cancer develops its own structure.

When cancer arises, it actually creates a specialized organ within an organ. It steals its own supporting cells and its own blood supply from its host organ to help it maintain its independent growth. Cancer cells are genetically unstable and can actually change the expression of some of their own genes, thereby releasing proteins that alter the noncancer cells in their environment to make them more supportive of cancer cell growth. In many cases, cancer cells develop the remarkable ability to break away from their original bases, float free in vascular channels, and set up a new growth in a distant organ. This is metastasis—the most feared development of a cancer.

As we live longer, our opportunity for acquiring cancer-inducing genetic mutations rapidly accelerates because the chromosomes that house genes become fragile with time. When we are young, our chromosomes avoid breakage because a specific shielding system, one of our molecular repair kits, keeps their ends well covered with a protective layer of protein. Those protective tips decay with time, particularly in cells that divide a great deal, such as the epithelial or lining cells of the ducts of the breast and prostate, the air passages of the lung, and the intestines.

Current dogma holds that the process of chromosome decay is gradual, but more recent data suggest that a single cell may undergo a cataclysmic event that renders its chromosomes susceptible to sudden fracture. When that untoward event occurs, the broken pieces randomly fuse with one another and copy themselves as chromosomes always do. Such fusions and copying of fragments of unpaired chromosomes are called unbalanced translocations. Once the process of fragmentation and extra chromosome production starts, it tends to self-perpetuate. At the sites where unpaired chromosomes are mashed into each other, certain genes critical to growth regulation may be amplified in number, deleted (erased), or mutated.

The mutations that cause cancer involve one or both of two classes of genes. The first includes genes that produce proteins that actively induce cancer when mutated because they foster continuous cell division. These are called dominant oncogenes, and the cancer-inducing proteins that they produce are called oncoproteins.

Oncoproteins work like jangling telephones. They send continuous signals to the cell nucleus to demand cell division. A single hypersignaling oncoprotein can actually cause the cell in which it arises to develop into a very large cancer. One role of smart drugs is to interact with oncoproteins and turn off their continuous jangling signals. But cancer cells are wily foes. Cancer is the result of mutations in regulatory genes, and cancer cells can continue to mutate, even in the face of drugs designed to kill them. These secondary mutations can prevent a smart drug from working. These enormously adaptable cancer cells are perfect examples of natural selection. The task of cancer researchers is to find enough smart drugs to overwhelm an individual cancer even though its oncogenes mutate further to avoid the executioner.

The second class of cancer-causing genes includes those that produce proteins that *prevent* cancer in their *non*mutated or normal state. They are called antioncogenes or tumor suppressor genes. It is bad news for a cell if a single copy of a gene is mutated, becomes a dominant oncogene, and the latter produces an oncoprotein that drives the cell to divide continuously. But just as bad is the loss of *both* copies of a tumor suppressor gene because tumor suppressor proteins may actually "sniff" along the DNA of cells and detect important mutations. When they find a segment of DNA that is in bad shape, such as the damage induced by a translocation, they signal the cell to commit suicide by turning its metabolism in a direction that sends the cell down a special death pathway.

When tumor suppressor protein is absent or in short supply, cells with a potential to cause cancer do not die. These cells accumulate and become actual cancers that can be very difficult to treat because they are relatively immortal. Further, since they do not die, the DNA remains in play to acquire more and more mutations until many dominant oncogenes are developed and more tumor suppressor genes are lost. The cell is in terrible shape from all this DNA damage, but it adapts to its own mutations until it has only one function left—that of dividing and surviving. This is a full-blown cancer cell. It is what probably occurred in one of the cells that lined Joan's breast milk duct.

Leukemias like Mario's and most sarcomas like Ken's gastrointestinal stromal tumor start in a different and more subtle way that is neither age nor time dependent. A single cell in Mario's bone marrow developed a reciprocal translocation between two unpaired chromosomes. Two different chromosomes literally snapped off a piece and swapped the broken-off pieces with each other. That sort of accident probably happens more than we know. When it does, the cell in which it occurs is usually sent down the death pathway by cellular executioners, the "sniffing" tumor suppressor proteins. Rarely, the swapping event puts a growth-inducing gene under the control of very strong gene expression machinery called a promoter. Many extra molecules of growth-inducing protein are then made. Or the growth-inducing gene may be mutated in the process, producing a hyperactive growth-inducing oncoprotein.

Finally, as in Mario's case, the translocation may produce a fusion gene made of two different genes. This may lead to a fusion protein that can induce many different genes to change the growth characteristics of the cell. Either way, the normal growth-regulating gene is turned into a dominant oncogene. The resulting stimulus to divide overwhelms the capacity of the sniffing proteins to detect the damaged DNA and send the affected cell down the death pathway. A massive proliferation of blood cells, all of which arise from the initially mutated cell, is the unfortunate result.

In Ken's case, the original mutation was very small. The chromosomes were intact when the first untoward event occurred. One specialized bowel cell called a Cajal cell, a nerve cell embedded in Ken's small intestine, developed a tiny mutation in one growth-regulating gene and turned it into a dominant oncogene. The mutated oncogene forced the cell to produce hyperactive growth-regulating oncoprotein, which in turn compelled the original cell to divide rapidly and grow into a sarcomatous cancer. As the sarcoma formed, additional mutations occurred, and other chromosomes began to exhibit breakage and unbalanced translocations. But the first event in Ken's cancer was just a very inopportune tiny error in one copy of one gene in one specialized nerve cell in his bowel.

We have learned a tremendous amount about cancer genetics, chemotherapy, and the future of smart drugs by studying and treating patients with leukemia like Mario and sarcoma like Ken. But epithelial cell cancers like Joan's breast cancer are much more frequent than leukemias or sarcomas. Our accomplishments in cancer research must therefore be measured by the progress that we gain in the prevention and treatment of epithelial cancers. To that end, we understandably focus cancer statistics on those diseases. If we are to reduce the burden of cancer, we must diminish the frequency or increase the cure rate of cancers like Joan's. The big four are breast cancer, prostate cancer, lung cancer, and colon cancer. These four cancers are our ultimate targets.

Can we prevent them? Though the medical literature and the popular press are regularly jammed with reports claiming that epithelial cancers might be prevented at least in part by dietary manipulations, the actual facts are less promising. Our DNA is under constant bombardment from solar radiation, natural and synthetic chemicals in food and air, and bacterial products in our intestines. The longer we live, the more mutations we sustain and the higher our likelihood of cumulative mutations that cause cancer.

This gloomy outlook notwithstanding, we could reduce cancer in the United States by 30 percent if we were to eliminate tobacco use. In fact, tobacco is such an enormous hazard that most other environmental cancer threats literally pale in significance when compared to it. Tobacco attacks DNA and causes dangerous cancers, particularly of the mouth, esophagus, lung, stomach, kidney, and bladder. The fact that it does not kill all smokers (and other tobacco users) suggests that good luck protects some of them, but luck runs out for at least half to two-thirds of the addicted victims. Smoking is like Russian roulette with three or four bullets in the cylinder of a six-shooter.

Diet has been a frenzied center of attention with respect to cancer. Dietary changes might reduce heart disease, but unfortunately they are at best of minimal benefit in preventing cancer. A long-term study recently supported by the National Institutes of Health has shown that reduction of dietary fat has marginal if any influence on heart and vascular disease or cancer. There is little or no evidence that emotional stress plays a causative role, either.

Cancer-inducing environmental hazards like asbestos contribute to only a tiny fraction of cancer cases. The fact is that we are at serious risk of unfavorable mutation merely by being on the planet for increasing amounts of time. Quitting smoking and avoiding excessive sun exposure increase your chances of not developing epithelial cell cancer, but only early death from another cause is guaranteed to prevent it. Time and mutation of DNA go hand in hand, and we are presently dealing with more than five hundred thousand invasive cancer deaths every year in the United States alone. There is some good news, however. Despite an increasing caseload (due to our growing senior population), total cancer deaths have peaked, and they began to decline in 2003. The attack on smoking, early cancer detection, and better treatments are beginning to work.

There is one other bit of very disquieting information about cancer burden for which we do not have a clear understanding. Overall cancer incidence data are misleading because they represent averages of an entire population of one country. They do not reveal the disparities in incidence of and mortality from cancer that are seen in our racial and ethnic minorities. These disparities are severe. The burden of cancer falls particularly heavily on African Americans, while Hispanics, Native Americans, and Alaskans have lower cancer incidences corrected for age. It seems that the expression of genes that modify the frequency and aggressive behavior of cancer may vary among races and ethnic groups. For example, an Icelandic company called Decode Genetics reported in 2006 that African Americans have twice the incidence of a gene on chromosome 8 that causes susceptibility to prostate cancer, and African American women tend to suffer from very aggressive forms of breast cancer. Other studies also suggest that there may be important environmental factors in certain groups that influence the frequencies of cancers. Regardless of cause, the obvious conclusion is that screening and effective preventive measures should target members of at-risk groups that are unusually susceptible to certain epithelial cancers and could benefit from such an effort.

It would be impossible to define an environmental cause of Mario's or Ken's cancer. That impossibility has not prevented families of cancer patients from mounting scores of investigations into power lines, water supplies, vaccinations, and air pollution. None of these avenues of research have been productive. But the majority of breast cancers like Joan's tumor are probably induced by a ubiquitous environmental product—estrogen.

The so-called epidemic of breast cancer observed in the past two decades can be ascribed to lifestyle changes that have in common a high exposure to estrogens. Estrogen is the likely culprit because most of the epidemic is due to an accumulation of estrogen-sensitive breast cancers in postmenopausal women—the very women who, like Joan, have been taking supplementary estrogen to control menopausal symptoms. And there are other clues. Breast cancer is more common in obese women than in thin women. Fat is a site of conversion of androgen to estrogen via the enzyme called aromatase. The disease is also seen more frequently in women who grew rapidly during adolescence or either had no pregnancies or delayed their pregnancies to their mid- to late thirties. All three circumstances exposed their breasts to a high level of estrogen or an increased number of estrogen production cycles. Japanese women have a low incidence of breast cancer in Japan, but among ethnic Japanese women living in the United States there is a higher incidence. The increased hazard could be ascribed to changes in selected foods, but it is more likely due to increased body weight, higher estrogen production, and higher odds of exposure to supplementary estrogens.

Excessive alcohol intake is a definite risk factor, and it is well known that alcohol inhibits the breakdown of estrogen in the liver and thereby causes the hormone to accumulate. The risk of alcohol confuses retrospective studies that suggest high folic acid (vitamin B9) intake reduces the incidence of breast cancer. Alcohol intake is associated with low folic acid consumption. Whether smoking influences breast cancer is somewhat disputed, although a recent study strongly suggests that it enhances the risk. To add to the confusion, a recent analysis suggests that regular ingestion of nonsteroidal anti-inflammatory drugs like ibuprofen (Advil or Motrin) also reduces the risk of breast cancer. It has not been well established how many women are nonsmokers and moderate drinkers, take supplementary vitamins, remain thin because they are athletic, and get sore joints and take ibuprofen. These intricate interactions complicate studies on the influence of habits and diet on cancer incidence.

The role of estrogen in breast cancer, however, is incontrovertible—so definite that the National Cancer Institute has conducted controlled prevention trials in women who are at high risk of the disease. High risk was defined as over age sixty, or in younger women, a strong family history of breast cancer. Joan, who is over sixty and has a family history, would have qualified for the trials. Half of the women who volunteered received tamoxifen, an estrogen blocker, for several years, and half did not. The incidence of breast cancer was much lower in the women given tamoxifen, and they did not suffer from a higher incidence of coronary artery disease or bone fracture, which are both thought to be consequences of estrogen insufficiency. Tamoxifen, however, acts as a *stimulant* of estrogen action in the uterus. Consequently, tamoxifen treatment can cause uterine cancer, a side effect that makes it less desirable as a breast cancer preventive.

Epithelial cancers would be even more frequent than they are were we not endowed with a DNA repair kit—a set of proteins that actually repair DNA mutations. Sadly, mutations may also attack repair kit genes. Some particularly unfortunate patients inherit repair kit mutations that cause a high incidence of cancer in their families. Younger patients with extensive family histories of breast or ovarian cancer may have inherited a normal and an abnormal copy (rather than two normal copies) of one of the two known breast cancer susceptibility genes called BRCA1 and BRCA2. They are both DNA repair genes. These unusual patients are at high risk of loss of the single remaining normal copy of the gene in one breast duct or ovarian epithelial cell. If such a loss occurs, the DNA of the affected cell accumulates damage because it cannot be repaired. All of the chromosomes break, elongate, increase in number, and mash into each other. Normal growth genes may then become activated and tumor suppressor genes lost. A malignant clone evolves into an invasive cancer. Prevention of breast cancer with tamoxifen is much less useful in these younger patients, particularly those with BRCA1 mutations, because the vast majority of their tumors are estrogen insensitive. Such patients, if identified early enough, may elect to have both breasts and ovaries removed to avoid the very high risk of breast or ovarian cancer with which they are confronted. The emotional trauma caused by this decision, known as a Hobson's choice, is well illustrated by Jessica Queller in a sobering self-report published in the *New York Times* in early 2005.

Given the high incidence and mortality of invasive cancer, it seems obvious that every effort should be devoted to early detection in order to permit effective local control. In fact, studies published in 2005 demonstrated that some of the improvement in breast cancer survival observed in the last three decades is due to the detection of these cancers while the tumor is small. But uncertainty and its handmaiden, controversy, dominate the early detection scene as well.

As you will read in Joan's story, a huge debate raged in the last decade about the value of screening mammography to detect early breast cancer. The issue has finally been settled in favor of mammography, but many experts still grumble. There are some who advocate the use of magnetic resonance imaging (MRI) as a supplement to mammography in breast cancer screening. But even the greediest imaging entrepreneur would have to agree that this hideously expensive test would be of little added value in women with a standard risk of contracting the disease. A 2004 study of very high-risk women (those with familial breast cancer or BRCA gene mutations), however, showed that the combination of MRI and mammography was superior to either one alone. For such patients, MRI supplementation of mammography is probably warranted despite the cost.

Contrary views of cancer screening are not limited to mammography. Much of the controversy is well documented in H. Gilbert Welch's book titled *Should I Be Tested for Cancer?* The prostate-specific antigen or PSA test, a blood test widely used in men over fifty to detect early prostate cancer, has severe critics as well. The national investment in the PSA test is huge. Due to false positives, many uncomfortable and occasionally risky biopsies of the prostate are performed without proven benefit. Also, many cases are missed because of false negatives. PSA screening probably detects prostate cancer in an earlier phase of the disease, but whether it saves lives is hotly debated. Most primary physicians utilize the PSA test in their practices despite the fact that the risk-benefit ratio is not completely established.

In 2005, Welch published a highly controversial paper on melanoma screening. Welch contends that the intensive screening for melanoma that has been the practice for the past decade has had no impact whatsoever on the death rate from melanoma. The new cases that have arisen from the screening are probably tumors that would not have become widespread. Welch's conclusions have released a storm of protest from dermatologists (who do the biopsies) and from the American Cancer Society. Careful skin examination should be part of a regular primary care program, but the value of screening clinics for melanoma is still under debate.

Screening for colon cancer is another contentious issue. The least expensive approach is a simple test for blood in the stools. But false negatives abound, particularly if the physician relies on a single stool examination, because many cancers of the colon do not bleed regularly. If blood testing in the stool is to be at all reliable, the patient must serially collect and test several daily samples. Even then, the test is not very robust. There are also many false positives because blood may appear in the stool for unrelated reasons such as hemorrhoids.

Colonoscopy is thought to be the best screening test, particularly because premalignant polyps can be detected and removed with that technique.

The test thus provides both early detection and prevention, but it is very expensive. Nonetheless, it is now offered to Medicare and Medicaid recipients, and almost all private insurers cover it as well. It provides an excellent living for endoscopists, but whether it saves enough lives to justify the cost depends on your view of appropriate health care spending. In a health care system such as ours, in which rationing is effectively based on wealth and employee fringe benefits, very expensive screening tests are usually reserved for the fortunate. Colonoscopy may be an unusual exception.

Then there is screening for lung cancer. Some experts advise an annual spiral computerized axial tomography (CAT) scan of the chest for patients at risk who have finally stopped smoking and appropriately fear the onset of lung cancer. This highly sensitive X-ray test can detect very small lesions (commonly called nodules) in the lungs. If a nodule is detected and is small (less than a centimeter or one-half an inch), it can be followed with serial examinations until the radiologist is confident that it is not growing. If it seems to be growing or is larger than a centimeter, a thoracic surgeon can remove it. The concept is reasonable because lung cancer is only curable if detected early and removed. But the cost to society could be tremendous. Though some hospitals offer the test for two to three hundred dollars, others are much more expensive. We currently await the final results of a large trial that is examining whether an annual spiral CAT scan can reduce deaths from lung cancer compared to screening with ordinary and far less expensive chest X-rays. In the meantime, based on preliminary data, if I had been a heavy smoker, I would ask for the test and hope my health insurance company would pay for it. If not, I would try to pay for it myself.

With respect to childhood lymphoblastic leukemia like Mario's, there is no evidence that early detection makes a difference in outcome. There are also no data to suggest that survival of a gastrointestinal stromal tumor like Ken's would be improved by early detection unless the tumor presented as a single well-encapsulated tumor that could be entirely removed by surgery. Since the early stages of the tumor rarely cause symptoms, early detection is very unusual. Neither leukemia nor gastrointestinal stromal tumor occurs at high enough frequency in the population to warrant large-scale screening.

If cancer control through prevention and screening is very difficult to achieve, treatment options must be extended. Surgery and local radiation therapy are the mainstays of treatment of local disease, but, as illustrated by the three cases in this book, cancer can be widespread at the moment of diagnosis. In the past forty years, we have relied on highly toxic carpet-bombing combination chemotherapy to try to blast the DNA of widespread cancer cells into oblivion. In some cancers, such as Mario's, and to a certain extent, Joan's, we have been successful. But most of the common epithelial cancers like lung, gastrointestinal, and prostate cancer and most of the sarcomas are quite resistant to the carpet-bombing approach, and toxicity is a major stumbling block.

Cancers like childhood leukemia, Hodgkin's lymphoma, cancer of the breast, cancers of the testis and the ovary, colorectal cancer, and many cancers of the head and neck have been successfully managed with the carpet-bombing approach of combination chemotherapy. The concept of the treatment is based on the selective toxicity exerted by antibiotics on infectious diseases. For example, severe infections with bacteria resistant to single antibiotics may be arrested by combinations of antibiotics that attack the organisms in different pathways of their metabolism. Meanwhile, some of the antibiotics may also be toxic to certain vital organs like the kidney. The hope is that cancer cells will be more vulnerable than normal cells to the toxic drugs.

Combination chemotherapy utilizes a group of broadly active compounds. Some inhibit DNA synthesis; some directly prevent cell division; others cause DNA to be chemically altered and therefore unable to copy itself. This alerts the "sniffing" proteins that detect damaged DNA and send the injured cell down a metabolic pathway that inexorably ends in death. Of course, the price of the attack is very high because of toxicity. Furthermore, the entire approach may fail because in many cancers the sniffing protein genes are mutated. Therefore, the combination of drugs is always chosen with an eye toward side effects and with more than a little expectation of failure.

There are many forms of toxicity. A particular carpet-bombing drug may mainly injure the gastrointestinal tract, the normal bone marrow, the nervous system, the kidney, the heart, or the pancreas. The oncologist tries to choose members of a combination, each of which evinces a different type of organ-specific nastiness in order to avoid "piling on" drugs of similar toxicity to a single organ or system.

There are both immediate and long-term toxic menaces. The immediate effects almost always include hair loss, fatigue, low blood cell counts, and nausea and vomiting; these are usually tolerable with supportive care. But the long-term effects can include irreversible damage to nerves, the heart, and the kidney. Some of the drugs may actually cause leukemia many years after they are administered. These are substantial risks, and the risks are not balanced by a high success rate in conditions such as lung, gastrointestinal, and brain cancer and invasive melanoma. This is why some critics believe that little progress has been made since we declared war on cancer in the 1970s and that we must set limits on health expenditures for fatal diseases. The controversy may help explain why unproven alternative or complementary therapies comprise a multibillion-dollar industry.

Clearly we do need alternatives to the carpet-bombing of cancer. We require drugs like penicillin that target the precise pathways that cancer cells adopt to assure their survival. These are the smart drugs—drugs that are screened for activity against a known single target, a protein on which cancer cells with very limited metabolic repertoires depend. That same protein may not be absolutely required by normal cells because the latter have much more redundancy of their metabolic pathways. Chromosome damage and gene loss limit the options for cancer cells, forcing them to rely on very few pathways for survival. That is their Achilles' heel. The task is to identify that lifeline and cut it. Though we need narrowly targeted smart drugs to defeat cancers and to reduce the toxicity of treatment, their discovery represents a technical challenge and a very expensive investment by grantors, academic research centers, and the pharmaceutical industry.

Hope that smart drugs might become available in a relatively short time came to me in the late 1970s and early 1980s when I learned of remarkable experiments carried out by my colleagues, Robert Weinberg at Massachusetts Institute of Technology and Philip Leder at Harvard Medical School. In 1979, Weinberg and his coworkers extracted DNA from a clone of mouse cancer cells and forced that DNA into a clone of normal mouse cells. The normal cells became cancer cells. The experiment proved that aberrant genes, now called dominant oncogenes, could cause cancer.

Three years later, Weinberg's laboratory obtained similar results in human cancer lines and also revealed the startling discovery that a human cancer such as bladder cancer could result from a very small point mutation in a normal gene that produces one of many growth-promoting proteins known as ras. The mutation in the ras gene that causes bladder cancer is so small that its only result is a single DNA base change in one copy of the two ras genes. The consequence is substitution of one building block amino acid for another in a protein that contains 171 amino acids. But such a change, while having no effect on the *amount* of the ras protein in the cell, markedly increases its *biological activity* and turns it into an oncoprotein called H-ras that causes unbridled growth of the mutated bladder epithelial cell and hence cancer. Clearly a drug that would interfere with the function of such an aberrant oncoprotein could cure the cancer with little or no toxicity because the malignancy entirely depends on that one oncoprotein for its survival, and normal cells do not require the hyperactive pathway.

Leder's experiment involved raising mice in which he had inserted new genes. Earlier he had been a discoverer of a chromosomal translocation in a human lymphoma that causes overproduction of myc, a growth regulatory protein. Its overproduction causes the lymphoma. When Leder forced mice to overproduce myc throughout their bodies, they developed lymphomas, but some also developed breast cancer. Then Leder forced the mice to overexpress an H-ras gene. They all developed breast cancer very quickly. A few years later, high myc expression and H-ras expression were found in many human epithelial cancers including breast cancer.

Weinberg's and Leder's discoveries ignited a firestorm of research aimed at discovery of the essential genetic changes that characterize the major cancers. Academic laboratories and pharmaceutical companies with strong research bases and millions of potential small molecules began to develop drug discovery programs based on assays of the activities of the particular oncoproteins that drive the cancer process. The goal was the production of smart antibodies or smart pills that would interfere with the precise pathways that cancer cells adopt to assure their survival and would force their destruction. The stories of Mario, Joan, and Ken tell how that progress was made.

# Mario's Story

# CHAPTER ONE

# The First Hours

That late Saturday afternoon in early May 1999 was gray and cold, and the emergency room at Children's Hospital in Boston was becoming hectic as it filled with the pediatric overflow of neighborhood health centers and private practice offices already closed for the day. Mothers lugging their sick children along with healthy siblings crammed into cubicles to talk to the triage nurse, the gatekeeper who would decide whether a child would languish in the reception area for most of the evening as a low-priority case or be deemed sick enough to come into the emergency area itself to wait in a cramped bed space for the first available physician. The mothers didn't complain. This was just one of the many nights some of them regularly spent in that well-worn reception space. Several were single mothers of a clutch of children. The whole family accompanied the sick one to spend the evening watching TV, guzzling soft drinks, and waiting for a doctor. This is the health care system for the uninsured. But overstressed urban teaching hospitals serve inconvenience with equal opportunity. The parents and children of the well-to-do languished as well, if they were deemed healthy enough to wait.

Mario, a nineteen-month-old, his mother, Flavia, and her mother-in-law had already spent most of a horrible afternoon in a pediatrician's office across the street. There, numbed with fear and shock, Flavia had been told to take Mario directly to the emergency room for immediate admission to the hospital.

She and her husband, Walter, were just barely keeping their heads above water. They were both immigrants, albeit from upper-middle-class Italian and Austrian families. Flavia's father was the regional manager of an express delivery company based in Milan. Walter's father was a successful manufacturer in Vienna. Flavia and Walter had yearned to be educated in the United States. Flavia wanted to become a commercial artist and Walter a marketing manager. They met in a community college in New York and shortly thereafter began to live together in Boston, where they started their careers. They married, and Flavia became pregnant. Mario's birth was difficult and resulted in mild nerve injury to his right arm, but he slowly recovered. Flavia actually brought him as a neonate to Children's Hospital for an evaluation of his arm, never dreaming that she would soon be spending months living there with her son.

The first year and a half of their new parenthood went reasonably well. Flavia has a creative flair for her work, and her list of private clients was growing. Walter had a harder time finding what he wanted, but just two weeks before the fateful visit to the pediatrician, he had landed a job with benefits, including health insurance, in the marketing department of a local manufacturer.

Around the time that Walter had started his new job, Mario was showing signs of not feeling well. He had no appetite, and walking appeared to exhaust him. After an hour or so of his usual careening around the family's small condominium, he would tire and be forced to rest. He also had a runny nose and a cough that wouldn't go away. Flavia began to take his temperature frequently. Sometimes he had a low-grade fever and would sleep for hours during the day.

For a while, Flavia and Walter thought Mario just had a stubborn virus. But the lack of appetite bothered them. Flavia took Mario to the pediatrician's office, where the nurse practitioner examined him carefully. Mario appeared fine. He looked healthy. Confident in the nurse practitioner, the pediatrician spent only a few minutes with Mario. She suggested acetaminophen (Tylenol) for the intermittent fever.

A week or two later, Flavia and Walter noticed scattered red spots on Mario's legs. This time, the pediatrician examined Mario and saw the spots, which measured less than an eighth of an inch in diameter. The doctor concluded that they represented a rash that often accompanies a viral infection. Again, she advised Tylenol for the fever, and she told Flavia to bring Mario back if anything new turned up.

What turned up was Walter's mother. She took one look at her grandson and bundled him up for another trip to the pediatrician's office. While Mario slept in his mother's lap, the grandmother demanded a blood test. When the nurse objected, she insisted on the test immediately. The nurse relented, did a finger stick on a howling Mario, and disappeared. A few minutes later, she reappeared looking haggard and disconcerted.

"We had trouble with the machine," she lied. "We'll have to repeat the test."

Again the finger stick. Again Mario's torrent of tears. Again the wait.

The pediatrician then appeared and said, "You have to go to Children's Hospital and be admitted immediately. I will call the emergency room and tell them to make sure you see an emergency physician right away while you wait for a bed to become available."

"But why?" Flavia asked.

"Keep your energy as much as you can, because you are going to need it," Mario's doctor responded. "The senior pediatrician in this practice is going to meet you in the emergency room as soon as he can and explain everything to you, but you must get over there immediately." With that terrifying warning, the doctor returned to her other patients.

Somehow Flavia absorbed the instructions. She knew she had to hold Mario close and carry him across the street. She blocked out the implications of her pediatrician's instructions so that she could make that short journey. Even her mother-in-law was silent. Grimly they made their way through the throng of sick and not-so-sick children in the reception area and were waved immediately into the emergency room to wait again. Walter was summoned from his new job as soon as the trio had settled in the cramped room. Flavia sat in a chair with Mario sleeping on her lap.

Flavia thought she was dreaming, but she remembers the details of the scene vividly. She recalls the pediatrician in charge of the practice entering the cramped space. "He was so tall and so skinny. He brought in a chair and turned it around so he could sit and lean forward on the back, and he didn't beat around the bush. He just said, 'Mario has leukemia.'" As she listened to the pediatrician, Flavia thought she had been struck down by fate.


The origin of the word *leukemia* is Greek. *Leukos* means "white" and *haima* means "blood." *Leukemia* means "white blood."

There are several classes of childhood leukemia based on the cell of origin. The most common class or type arises in lymphocytes, the small, round white cells that circulate in the blood, lymphatic channels, and lymph nodes and are responsible in part for the control of infection by bacteria, viruses, parasites, and fungi.

In children, the most common subset of lymphocytic leukemia is acute lymphoblastic leukemia (ALL). It usually starts when a single, immature lymphoblast (the most immature precursor of lymphocytes) begins to grow uncontrollably in the bone marrow. Sometimes an enormous mass of cells derived from the original cell fills the marrow, the spleen, the lymph nodes, and the blood. In unusual ALL cases, so many leukemic cells accumulate in the blood that it actually turns white; hence the disease's name. But in most cases, the leukemic cells replace the marrow, where they prevent normal blood cell production and do not accumulate excessively in the circulation.

There are two major subsets of ALL based on the type of lymphocyte in which the leukemia arises. The most common is B-cell ALL. The B-lymphocyte is the producer of antibodies. Less common is T-cell ALL. T-lymphocytes directly kill viruses, fungi, and certain bacteria such as the tuberculosis bacillus.

When Walter heard the diagnosis, he began to laugh and couldn't stop. "You're kidding—what are you talking about?" It wasn't Walter's usual laugh, though. The laugh rose hysterically. Suddenly he turned very pale and fell totally silent for a few seconds. Then Walter collected himself and took charge. "Okay, what do we do now?"

When Walter asked that question, Flavia awakened from her dreamlike state. Mario's life was not over today. She had to take action, come up with a plan. Through her desperation, she heard the pediatrician refer to two kinds of leukemia and mention that neither variety is great, but it is much better to learn you have one than the other—the "good" leukemia and the "bad" leukemia, she seemed to hear. She decided that Mario had to have the "good" leukemia. She clutched at that idea and repeated "good leukemia" like a mantra.

The hospital's prosaic boredom, discomforts, and a sense of some organized flow began to replace the terror in her heart. The academic medical center parade of doctors and their attendant medical students began. The intern, followed by the emergency medicine resident, followed by the resident in charge of the house staff on the oncology service; the attending (supervisory) emergency physician; the oncology attending and first-year oncology trainee (the fellow); the intensive care house staff;

the attending in intensive care; and all the nurses, medical students, and ward secretaries associated with them marched through Flavia's life over the next twenty-four hours. Keeping Mario either on her lap or next to her in a transportable bed, she tried to listen and kept repeating "good leukemia."

While Mario was still in the emergency room, several medical staff attempted to draw blood and start an intravenous drip of fluid, but Mario's veins were recalcitrant. Then an expert IV nurse came in with a basket of what looked like Roman candles: needles encased in tubes of plastic. Mario screamed when he saw her, but she eventually succeeded in starting the IV, although leaving bruises. Next came the long trip through X-ray and on to the oncology service, where Mario was put to bed in a room opposite the nurses' station, a site of constant noisy activity but the safest place on the ward because of its proximity to the nurses. Sometime near a restless dawn, Mario was transferred to the intensive care unit. A bed had finally become available. Flavia remembers one particularly kind nurse who saw she was exhausted and asked her if she wanted to lie on the bed with Mario while they were both rolled through the corridors and down the elevator to the unit. She might have fallen asleep for a moment on that voyage.

By this time, Walter had gone home to do an Internet search and read everything he could about leukemia. He prepared himself to call Flavia's client list of commercial art firms and let them know that her presentations would be indefinitely delayed. Walter's mother went with him.

Flavia stayed with Mario and the medical entourage. Out of the crowd of doctors stepped Scott Armstrong, a first-year fellow in oncology. She remembers their first meeting in precise detail. Flavia felt as though she had been drifting in a turbulent sea, drowning in the unexpected wreck of her life. Suddenly a life ring was flung to her from the fog. Holding the rope was Scott. In his inexperience, Scott had no idea of the importance of that moment, but he saved Flavia from profound depression.

Scott Armstrong is an Oklahoma boy. He is not physically big, but he is determined and has a fine mind to boot. Early on, he knew he was destined for science. Chemistry and math fascinated him in high school, and he had good teachers who encouraged him. At the University of Oklahoma, he had a chance to work in relating the latest aspect of molecular biology to the blood-clotting system. The experience convinced Scott to become a physician scientist committed to a career involving blood-related cancers. That way, he could explore his passion for science and help people at the same time. He entered the M.D./Ph.D. program at University of Texas Southwestern Medical School. Scott worked in the lab of two of the best biomedical research trainers in the business, Michael Brown and Joseph Goldstein, physicians who had won a Nobel Prize for their work on cholesterol metabolism. Scott wasn't particularly interested in cholesterol, but he knew he would learn to be a scientist in that laboratory. Hematological (blood-related) oncology could wait until he completed his residency training.

During his schooling, Scott realized that he wanted to work with sick children. He related to them as friends, wanted to help them, and found his soothing, confident manner was a comfort to agonized parents whose children faced death. He applied for postgraduate pediatric training at Children's Hospital, where I was chief of pediatrics. I received a brief letter about him from Joe Goldstein. The last sentence was, "Just take him, you won't regret it."

My residency program did not regret it. Scott was an excellent addition to the house staff. Cheerful on little sleep and enormously competent, he set a fine record on every rotation. The combined Children's Hospital and Dana-Farber Cancer Institute's program is prestigious, and competition for slots in its hematology oncology fellowship is intense. Scott made the cut in the first round of decisions. He started his first year of fellowship in the July prior to Mario's May admission.

His first patient as a fellow was an eight-month-old infant (by medical definition, infants are children younger than one year old) with leukemia. Scott was particularly challenged by the very rare mixed-lineage leukemias he saw in infants. He learned that older children with the usual ("good") form of acute childhood leukemia (acute lymphoblastic leukemia, or ALL) do very well today. Eighty to eighty-five percent of them are cured of the disease. Scott mastered the art of differentiating that kind from the less common one, acute myeloblastic leukemia (AML), which arises in larger white cells designed to attack and ingest bacteria. This is the "bad" leukemia; its response to treatment, though reasonable, is not as good as the response of children with ALL. Until twenty-five years ago, every such child died; today, about half of children with AML remain disease-free.

Scott introduced himself to Mario's exhausted and frightened mother, speaking warmly and carefully to her. He had already examined Mario, who did not have remarkable physical findings other than the red spots on his legs, and he knew that Mario had a low platelet count. Platelets are responsible for initiating the clotting of blood; hence the small hemorrhagic red spots on Mario's legs. Mario was somewhat anemic as well, but it was the white blood cell count of nearly one million per cubic millimeter of blood (normal is about five thousand) that had prompted the emergency admission and transfer to the intensive care unit. It was difficult to decide whether the swarm of malignant white cells were ALL or AML cells. They formed the classic picture of mixed-lineage leukemia (MLL) seen in infants. Flavia, who was praying for "good" rather than "bad" leukemia, was going to have to face that her son might have a third kind: "terrible" leukemia.

Scott knew he had to be careful in his initial conversations with Flavia. She was alone, exhausted, and extremely vulnerable. Whatever he told her would have to be backed with solid evidence and not conjecture. She immediately pressed him: "Is this the good leukemia?" His answer was that he could not be certain until other laboratory tests were concluded, but in any case, the immediate risk was not the type of leukemia but the very high white blood cell count. The level of leukemia cells in Mario's blood would have to be reduced immediately, for several reasons. The most pressing was that leukemic cells tend to clump. Sticky, sugary proteins on their surfaces, a general characteristic of cancer cells, make them adhere to blood vessel walls and to one another. The result is a plug that can block a major blood vessel and cause a stroke. Mario might not recover from such a crisis. The leukemic cells might also die more rapidly than normal cells. When they die, they burst and release their contents—huge amounts of potassium and phosphorus—into the circulation. The sudden release of that load might stop Mario's heart.

Scott's first action was to perform an exchange transfusion, a procedure in which Mario's blood, with its swarming leukemic cells, would be removed and replaced with normal blood. That would lower his leukemic cell count and avert a crisis. As soon as that exchange occurred, Scott promised to deal with the exact type of leukemia and propose a treatment.

Flavia listened and signed the consent forms after reading them cursorily, but her mind was almost blank. (So much for informed consent under stress.) She had only three thoughts: Would Mario survive all this? Would he finally become well? Would she have him back again? She couldn't say she really understood Scott's approach, but she trusted him on sight.

Scott mobilized the specialized staff, and the exchange procedure started at once. Leaving Mario in the competent hands of the intensive care people, Scott called Lewis Silverman, a staff physician at Children's Hospital and the Dana-Farber Cancer Institute and an assistant professor at Harvard Medical School, to go over the next steps in what would turn out to be a two-year effort to save Mario.

CHAPTER TWO

# The Plan

When called by Scott to develop a plan for Mario, Lew Silverman was already certain that Mario's leukemia would present a major clinical challenge. The cancer was not the ordinary ALL of childhood. Silverman was confident that detailed laboratory studies would show that Mario had the mixed-lineage leukemia (MLL) of infancy, even though he was older than most of the patients diagnosed with that perilous, rare disorder. Scott had not seen much MLL, which comprises only about 10 percent of all cases of leukemia in childhood. And childhood leukemia represents only 1 percent of the total cancer incidence in the United States. An oncologist, even a pediatric oncologist, encounters few cases of MLL in a lifetime unless he or she is associated with a cancer center with a very large referral base of pediatric cases. Only a handful of such centers are in the United States, and the program at Children's Hospital and Dana-Farber is one of them.

Nonetheless, Scott had been thinking hard about MLL ever since he had seen a case in his first month of fellowship. He had several persistent questions about the disease: What is the genetic basis of the disorder? What DNA mutations are responsible? And would detailed knowledge of the mutations and their effects offer better options for treatment? He had already decided to work in the laboratory of the late Stanley J. Korsmeyer, a well-known researcher at Dana-Farber who had discovered one of the fundamental truths about cancer. Twenty years before Mario had been admitted to Children's Hospital, Korsmeyer had convinced the cancer community of what then seemed to be a new concept: cancer often results from mutations in DNA that prevent cells from dying. The standard dogma at the time (that cancer is always caused by mutations that force cells to divide too rapidly) was oversimplified. Korsmeyer's studies showed that many normal cancer cells are endowed with "sniffing" monitor proteins that crawl along the DNA and detect unfavorable mutations that have not been repaired. If those proteins locate an unrepaired mutation, they send a signal that starts the cell down a death pathway. The trail ends in a release of enzymes that crunch up the cell's nucleus, turning it into a prune pit.

Such cell death can actually be good for the body. DNA is constantly bombarded by mutagens, the invading chemicals and radiations that change (mutate) genes. Most of those invaders arise from natural chemical reactions in our internal environment. We operate our own private sewage plant in our lower intestines, where bacteria are constantly growing and producing all kinds of chemicals: some solid, some liquid, and some gas. Many of those chemicals can seriously damage the DNA packaged in the chromosomes, which in turn are stuffed into our cells' nuclei. Added to the mutagen stew are external contaminants such as radiation from outer space, tobacco smoke, gasoline emissions, and more. Cells with mutated genes may divide and multiply endlessly, a defining characteristic of cancer. The sniffing proteins ward off cancer by sending mutated cells down the death pathway. If the genes that form those sniffing proteins are mutated, cancer is a regular consequence.

At the time he met Mario, Scott was still a first-year fellow and his job was to care for patients. He had to make a firm diagnosis, and he needed a treatment plan that might work, despite lacking all the information he wanted. Fortunately, Silverman also was especially interested in infant leukemia, because it seemed to be one of the last leukemias recalcitrant to chemotherapy.

Huge strides had been made in the management of ALL, the most common cause of childhood leukemia. That's why Flavia and one of Mario's pediatricians had called it the good leukemia. And even treatment for AML, the so-called bad leukemia, had come a long way. But before Silverman and his mentor, Stephen Sallan, a professor and the leader of the pediatric oncology clinical program at Children's Hospital and Dana-Farber—together with a group of Dutch pediatric oncologists, a large German team, and colleagues at St. Jude's Children's Research Hospital in Memphis—had established an international trial in 1997 of a new treatment program, pediatric cancer doctors adjudged MLL (mixed-lineage leukemia) virtually unmanageable. Almost all afflicted infants died.

Sallan had begun to attack the problem in the early 1980s on a necessarily small scale. Why were the infants with MLL, unlike the vast majority of children with standard ALL and even the small majority with AML, so resistant to effective treatment? Were the MLL-afflicted infants simply unable to handle anticancer drugs or did the MLL cells have one or more differences that required an additional treatment drug?

Lacking evidence on anticancer drug metabolism in infants, Sallan, along with Silverman, who had just completed his first year of fellowship, elected to add to the treatment a drug that had not previously been used in the management of MLL. The drug, cytosine arabinoside, or AraC, has been around for decades and had been employed largely to treat AML. MLL cells have some of the characteristics of leukemic lymphoblasts, but they also have some of the characteristics of leukemic myeloblasts (cells associated with AML). Since AraC acts so effectively against acute myeloblastic leukemia, the researchers decided to try it for MLL. Slowly and painfully, Silverman began to collect a total of eleven newly diagnosed patients with MLL from around the United States and Canada. In 1985, he and Sallan devised a protocol in which they added AraC to the standard regimen for ALL. Thirteen years later, Silverman tentatively reported that almost half of the MLL patients enjoyed prolonged disease-free survival with the new protocol. The results were encouraging, but the number of patients was much too small to provide certainty. While that small trial was in progress, Dutch colleagues developed excellent evidence that MLL cells have a curious protein on their surfaces that can actually pump the antileukemic drug AraC into them. The MLL cells use that pump for other purposes, but the Dutch data clearly provided a rationale for intensive AraC treatment.

As this direct chemical evidence confirmed the clinical findings, the consortium of European and North American investigators began to attack MLL in earnest. The collaboration required extensive tolerance. The Europeans had their ideas about the optimal protocol. The Americans had theirs. The groups compromised, amalgamating the best of both.

The much larger trial continues even now as I write, and it looks promising. As of 2004, 320 infants, most of whom had documented MLL, had been enrolled. The overall survival without relapse was 50 percent.

For those with documented MLL, it was nearly 40 percent. This is a huge improvement, and it confirms Silverman's preliminary results, but more research is definitely needed.

Scott knew much of the background about MLL treatment research in May 1999, but he needed a precise diagnosis of Mario's condition. He and Silverman first gazed at the child's cells carefully under a microscope. They suspected MLL because they could see features of lymphoblasts and myeloblasts in the stained smear. But they had to gather more evidence from a fluorescence-activated cell sorter, a machine that uses monoclonal antibodies to separate various kinds of cells.

That machine's origins stem from work done more than twenty-five years ago. In 1979, George Kohler and César Milstein, two basic scientists at the University of Cambridge in the United Kingdom, developed a method that could grow a clone of millions of cells that produce a single antibody. Those researchers deservedly received a Nobel Prize just five years later, in 1984. They never patented their discovery, believing that the fruits of science should be available to all without restriction. Soon afterward, different monoclonal antibodies became commercially available around the world. By using such antibodies, doctors can now distinguish different leukemias, diagnose the origin of many other cells in health and disease, and treat quite a few illnesses (from various cancers to inflammatory diseases like rheumatoid arthritis). The new method proved quite reliable and much more objective than the art of diagnosing various leukemias by examining the appearance of cells under microscopes.

Scott and Silverman could not be sure about Mario's diagnosis until the technicians could come in the next day and analyze Mario's cells in a cell sorter with monoclonal antibodies. The doctors decided to delay having a complete discussion with Flavia until they could confirm the results and until Walter was available to support her.

The extraordinarily high white blood cell count also gave Scott and Silverman plenty to do over the next twelve to twenty-four hours. The exchange transfusion ongoing in the ICU was only step one. They would have to give Mario a low dose of doxorubicin (Adriamycin), a good chemotherapeutic drug, to cut down on the population of cancer cells in his blood. And they would have to be sure he was well hydrated so that he could urinate out all the potassium and phosphorus that would come from the dying leukemic cells.

Scott returned to Flavia after his meeting with Silverman and told her the plan was to take things slowly and in phases during the coming day, using that period to lower Mario's risk of a crisis. Meanwhile, he suggested that Flavia should try to sleep a bit. A detailed conference would follow the next day.

Flavia instinctively trusted Scott. She fell asleep for short periods in the midst of worrying about the day to come.

Scott doesn't remember if he slept at all that night. He checked frequently on the status of Mario's exchange transfusion and also dealt with new patients. On his visits to Mario, he saw that Flavia was usually awake. She sat by Mario's bedside, fingering her rosary beads.

Come morning, Scott was energized by the appearance of the technicians as they prepared to study Mario's cells in the cell sorter. When the results came in, he saw that they were as he and Silverman had predicted. They bore markers of both lymphoid and myeloid lineage; that is, they were of mixed lineage. The diagnosis of MLL was close to being confirmed. Absolute confirmation would have to await a more complex investigation of the leukemic cells' chromosomes to determine if they were normal. In this test, dividing cells would be squashed on a glass slide to break their nuclei and spread the chromosomes. Then technicians would stain those to detect any translocation.

Translocations—the result of abnormal pairing of chromosomes during cell division—frequently appear in leukemic white blood cells. Leukemia can erupt because on rare occasions an accident occurs in one of the millions of cells in the bone marrow. Two different chromosomes break apart, and the resulting pieces fuse incorrectly to make two new, abnormal chromosomes. In the case of MLL, such translocations cause the development of an abnormal gene, which produces an abnormal protein that drives the leukemic cells to divide and avoid the death pathway.

Every year, doctors learn of about four hundred children worldwide who end up with translocations that cause MLL. That was the case with Mario. Scott would become involved in determining more about the science of MLL upon entering Korsmeyer's lab a few months later. If the answer could be found, Scott knew he would be much closer to a good treatment plan for infant leukemia. That would enable him to give far more effective care to Mario.

For now, Scott needed to hold a meeting with Walter and Flavia to go over the next steps in treating their son. He had to be reasonably flexible because the final diagnosis was not in while he also had to begin teaching the parents about leukemia and its management. He expected a long, difficult discussion that would be quite emotional.

Before that all-important meeting, Flavia put her child in a rolling cart and pushed him to the elevator, down to the first floor, and into a peaceful garden that is part of Children's Hospital. The weather had turned warm that Sunday morning. "It was a beautiful day," Flavia recalled later. "I took his shoes off . . . I wanted to give him a feeling of grabbing energy." Then the two returned indoors.

A few minutes later, the meeting began in the room Flavia and Walter would come to call the "bad news room," because that was where they would hear news that always seemed threatening to Mario. Scott explained that Mario's leukemic cell count had been cut in half and was still falling as the result of the small dose of Adriamycin. The immediate crisis had been averted. Mario was no longer in danger of having a sudden stroke or heart attack. Scott began to talk slowly and gently about Mario's diagnosis. Mario had leukemia, the exact type to be determined. Chemotherapy treatment had to start at once, and Mario would have to stay in the hospital for a month or more to protect him from the toxicity of the treatment. For further evaluation of the extent of his disease, Mario also needed a bone marrow examination and a spinal tap. Flavia and Walter found the information almost overwhelming, and they signed myriads of consent forms without being entirely sure of the risks and benefits.

During that meeting, Scott purposely did not give them the entire, terrible story about MLL. He wanted them to have some time to adjust to what he was saying. The immediate tasks were to deliver the best possible therapy to Mario and to give him all the support he needed. His parents' morale would be the key.

At a second meeting, Scott began to explain the first one-month stage of therapy beyond the events that had already taken place in the ICU. The first job was to induce a remission, which simply means that the bone marrow and blood become microscopically free of leukemic cells, and levels of different normal components of blood—including red cells, platelets, and white cells (the germ eaters)—return to normal or near normal. Mario's medical team would accomplish this with a set of drugs that had been available for years. The group would administer the same doses of drugs using the same schedule that was used for every child regardless of ALL type. The details about these drugs will be described in a subsequent chapter.

As previously mentioned, Mario was given Adriamycin. Mario would also receive methotrexate, one of the first drugs found to be effective in leukemia treatment. It interferes with the synthesis of DNA. He would also receive an enzyme called asparaginase, which lowers the level of an amino acid, asparagine, in the blood and tissues. Asparagine is required by ALL cells to make their necessary proteins.

Finally, Mario would be treated with vincristine, which is derived from the periwinkle plant and prevents cells from dividing by interfering with the proteins that pull the chromosomes apart, and he would be given prednisone, a steroid modeled on the hormones of the adrenal gland because such hormones are known to kill leukemic lymphoblasts by sending them down the death pathway.

This array of compounds would form a multifaceted attack on leukemic cells. Scott and Silverman were confident Mario would go into remission with this virtual military assault from all sides.

Flavia and Walter understood the plan and the explanation of the drugs and their various side effects, such as hair loss, nausea and vomiting, and low blood counts, in a limited way. They gave their okay to Scott, and he began writing the orders and preparing to ask the nurses and pediatric residents to take over. The situation would focus on good care and attention to detail—and time and patience.

The nurses set up a cot for Flavia in Mario's room. She would barely leave the hospital for the next two months.

CHAPTER THREE

# Leukemia and Cancer Chemotherapy

As Scott Armstrong and Lew Silverman recounted to me their initial meetings with Mario and his parents, I could not help but reflect on my own first experiences in treating patients with childhood leukemia. When I was a new clinical associate at the National Cancer Institute (NCI) in Bethesda, Maryland, in 1956, I did not expect to save a single child or adult with any kind of widespread cancer at all. Though Mario's unusual type of leukemia still presents a difficult problem, the care of most patients with the disease has undergone a sea change in the past four decades.

The vast change for the better came about largely because Sidney Farber, an intensely complex visionary, declared a personal war against childhood leukemia. Only about five thousand cases of childhood leukemia arise annually in the United States. The number represents just 1 percent of the nation's cancer burden, but Farber hated every case and ended up devoting his life to trying to eradicate the disease.

I first heard Sidney Farber speak in 1953 during my second year of study at Harvard Medical School. The talk was a depressing, even sepulchral, lecture on childhood cancer—one that did not make the field attractive for doctors-to-be, even those who were incurable optimists. But Farber's passionate hatred of a disease that killed children in just a few months and left their parents in desperate grief, and his determination to find drugs that would cure patients, came through in the hour-long discussion.

Farber was looking for a magic bullet—a smart drug that would go straight to the problem, attacking the cancer cells in a child's body while causing the child as little harm as possible. Farber wasn't the first scientist to seek a smart drug to solve what might look like an unsolvable medical problem. Alexander Fleming's discovery of penicillin changed the face of medicine. The finding of penicillin in bread mold remains the paradigm of the unearthing of antibiotics and led to the broadly active carpet-bombing anticancer drugs.

Penicillin turned out to be a true smart drug. It attacks a specific molecule in the membrane of certain bacteria and has virtually no effect on human cells. Since its discovery, molds, metals, and soil samples from throughout the world, and plants, including herbs, trees, and even their barks, have provided hundreds of potential antimicrobial and anticancer agents. Artemesin, a derivative of a Chinese herb, with striking antimalarial activity, is one of the latest examples.

Pharmaceutical companies and government laboratories have screened thousands of natural substances searching for antibiotic and anticancer activity. Most of the substances that have emerged from the screens have very broad effects including inhibition of protein synthesis, breakage of cell membranes, damage to DNA, and prevention of cell division. Those pursued as antibiotics must be reasonably selective, meaning that their toxicity must be largely limited to microorganisms. Those with broader toxicity to animal cells are investigated as possible anticancer agents with the hope that cancer cells will be more vulnerable than normal cells to the toxic drug.


Farber had come from a hardworking Jewish family in Buffalo, New York, the third of fourteen children, many of whom became successful physicians. Farber sought training in Heidelberg, Germany, after his graduation from the University of Buffalo. In Heidelberg, he resolved to devote himself to medical research. He was admitted to the class of 1927 of Harvard Medical School (HMS), already committed to becoming a pathologist, and he never left. He rose to become a professor of pathology and one of the most distinguished cancer scientists in the world.

Back in the 1920s, Farber found some of the people at HMS inhospitable to Jews. The environment did not affect his overwhelming work ethic or his rise in the ranks of the faculty. He was soon appointed the chief of the pathology program at Children's Hospital, a famous but then antiquated Harvard teaching hospital. There he began to explore childhood leukemia.

He became fascinated by the similarity between what happens as leukemia progresses in the bone marrow where most blood cells are made and what occurs in the marrow when people become deficient in two of the B vitamins: vitamin B12 and folic acid (vitamin B9). In childhood leukemia, the marrow becomes filled with primitive lymphoblasts. These are the precursors of the normal lymphocytes that regulate immunity. But the leukemic lymphoblasts never mature to normal lymphocytes. They just keep dividing until they occupy the entire marrow space and drive out all the normal cells.

In the case of B12- and folic acid–deficient patients, vitamin-deficient blood-forming cells in the marrow also become arrested in their development and grow very large. These cells are called megaloblasts because they are big and primitive. After several months or years of severe vitamin B12 or folic acid deficiency, megaloblasts that cannot develop into normal blood cells dominate the marrow. Such vitamin-deficient patients experience a severely reduced production of normal blood cells including red cells, white cells, and platelets. This condition is known as pancytopenia.

Pancytopenic patients are profoundly anemic and therefore weak; they are easily infected; and they often bleed into the skin, the mouth, the gut, and the urine. These are precisely the symptoms of leukemia, the difference being that in leukemia malignant cells are found in the blood and throughout the body. But the damage to the patient created either by leukemia or by the vitamin deficiencies is very similar. In both conditions, the patients usually die of the results of pancytopenia.

Farber was particularly fascinated by research begun in the late 1920s that eventually led to the isolation, purification, and structural analysis of both vitamins. A few micrograms of vitamin B12 or 5 milligrams of folic acid rapidly normalize the marrow of deficient patients and completely correct the pancytopenia.

Farber had rodents with leukemia in his laboratory. He had treated them with the recently discovered adrenal hormone called cortisone. The leukemic cells disappeared but always came back. As soon as crude preparations of vitamin B12 and folic acid became available in the early 1940s, he treated the rats with the extracts—to no avail, but he remained convinced that leukemia might be due to an acquired form of vitamin deficiency. He needed more vitamins to test, and that is when he began a crucial collaboration with an immigrant from India, Yellapragada SubbaRow.

SubbaRow had come to HMS in 1923 to study for a Ph.D. in biochemistry after he received his first Ph.D. in tropical medicine from London University. To support himself, he worked as an orderly in one of the HMS teaching hospitals. In 1940, having risen to the rank of associate professor of biochemistry, SubbaRow left Harvard to assume the scientific directorship of what was then Lederle Laboratories (now subsumed by Wyeth Pharmaceuticals). There he began to modify the folic acid molecule in a search for new vitamin activities. That immediately attracted the attention of Farber, who wanted to test SubbaRow's modified folic acid compounds in normal and leukemic rats.

The two men maintained an active correspondence throughout the 1940s. Letters document the collaboration and show how their thinking slowly shifted from the search for a new vitamin to the realization that an antivitamin might actually work in leukemia. Farber first tested SubbaRow's new folic acid–like compounds in healthy animals. Initially the two men were disappointed. Most of the newly synthesized compounds had no activity, and those that did were not marrow stimulants but rather depressed the blood counts of normal animals. They actually induced pancytopenia.

Then Farber had a brilliant idea. Perhaps one or more of SubbaRow's synthetic compounds would kill experimental leukemic cells more than it would kill normal marrow cells. Farber treated rodents with experimental leukemia with the synthetic folic acid–like compounds (called analogues in the parlance of medicinal chemistry and antimetabolites in the language of nutrition). One analogue called aminopterin (the chemical name for the parent folic acid is pteropterin) proved particularly active in the rodent system. It destroyed the animal leukemia cells. It also played havoc with normal blood production and damaged the animals' intestines.

Farber and SubbaRow ascribed these side effects to dose and schedule of administration of a powerful vitamin antagonist, an antivitamin or antimetabolite. The cell is fooled by the appearance of the antimetabolite because its chemical structure looks so much like the real folic acid. Once the antimetabolite enters the metabolic pathway, it becomes stuck in one position and effectively blocks the stream of molecules that move down the pathway. Several years later, it was shown that the pathways that involve folic acid and vitamin B12 intersect and that the final product of both vitamins is DNA.

Though their knowledge of the dose range and toxicity of any anti-metabolite in humans was very incomplete, Farber, with support from SubbaRow and Lederle, decided to take the next momentous step: to test the most likely drug, aminopterin, or its first cousin—a drug called methotrexate—in children with ALL. That decision plunged the physi-cians and the patients into an uncharted sea. Though aminopterin and methotrexate seemed to be smart drugs because they block a metabolic pathway in cells, they were really not smart at all because they blocked an essential pathway that is required by *all* of the dividing cells in the body as well as by dividing cancer cells. That is why normal rats became pancytopenic and developed intestinal disorders when they received the drugs. Nonetheless, in 1946, Farber and his colleague, Louis K. Dia-mond, then the chief of hematology at Children's Hospital, forged ahead and treated sixteen children with ALL with the new drugs. The results were spectacular. Ten of them achieved complete remission, meaning there was no visible evidence of leukemia cells. Farber and Diamond's report, published in the *New England Journal of Medicine* in 1948, began the modern era of cancer chemotherapy with targeted (if not smart) drugs.

It is important at this juncture to reflect on the research experience in 1946 and compare it to clinical research in the twenty-first century. In 1946, these children were treated with an entirely experimental drug, a class of drug that had never before been given to humans. The children were too young to give informed consent. In fact, there was no formal consent process at all. The parents of the children seized the opportunity because they trusted their physician, Louis Diamond, and when they met Dr. Farber, they were awed. The "informed" consent was obtained orally based on the parents' understanding that their children were going to die; that these trusted doctors were trying to save them. Today, such a process would be totally unacceptable and might even lead to prosecution. It would certainly cause the removal of all National Insti-tutes of Health (NIH) grants, vilification in the medical literature, and, in some cases, in the public news media.

The change in our approach to informed consent in clinical research has its roots in World War II. The public and our political leaders were overwhelmed by revelations of the incredible brutality of Nazi physicians who experimented on concentration camp victims. Their behavior was so heinous that it shocked the world. But most believed that such behavior could never occur at home. Americans, full of a sense of their own rectitude, were only mildly disturbed in 1966 when Henry Beecher, a professor of anesthesiology at Harvard Medical School, published a now classic paper in the *New England Journal of Medicine* in which he pointed out that violations of the cardinal ethical principle of informed consent in clinical trials were much more frequent than either the public or the medical community realized. Six years later, the American public went into shock. In 1972, news broke that officers of the highly trusted U.S. Public Health Service, excellent physicians and devoted government employees, had since 1932 conducted an experiment on poor, black residents of Alabama who had syphilis. Without their knowledge or consent, penicillin treatment had been withheld from the patients when it became available in the late 1940s in order to follow the natural course of the disease. The outrage was enormous. Congress reacted predictably, and the first stages of a highly complicated set of procedures for the establishment of informed consent began to be promulgated.

There are still some problems, but the informed consent system is vastly improved since that important moment in 1946 when Farber and Diamond told the parents of children with leukemia that they would try an entirely untested therapy. There is no documented evidence that any of those parents understood the potential risks and benefits in any detail. They leapt for the treatment because they had no other hope. And Diamond and Farber were convinced that they were acting on behalf of the patients. In those early days of clinical research, the best protection of the patient was the moral sense of the physician scientist. Unfortunately, subsequent events demonstrated that moral instinct is an insufficient guardian. Almost all physicians believe that they are acting in the best interests of their patients even when neutral outside observers come to a totally different conclusion about the risk-to-benefit ratios. As is true of all other aspects of research, peer review is essential.

In the case of the Farber and Diamond experiment, the results for the patients and the physicians seemed quite marvelous. Acute lymphoblastic leukemia remissions lasting more than a few weeks had never before been observed. The report in the *New England Journal of Medicine* is now considered a classic in medicine. And the initial group of ten responders was temporarily overjoyed. Sadly, all of them relapsed within a year of their successful induction of remission, but Farber believed that this setback also represented a dose and schedule problem that he could solve with further trials. More drugs were needed. He was certain that he could find an approach that would hold the patients in remission.

As Farber set out in 1946 to do the first trials of aminopterin and methotrexate in the sixteen children, members of the Variety Club of Boston—consisting largely of owners of movie theaters—visited him to consider offering a large charitable donation for his work. His office was unprepossessing and his laboratory a dingy room in the basement of a century-old building hobbled by poor lighting, inadequate ventilation, and primitive equipment, but Farber was a towering presence. A tall, portly man, he wore a stiffly starched and spotless white coat buttoned from top to bottom. His face was pale, topped by black hair only slightly tinged with gray and interrupted by a black mustache and dark eyes. His voice was soft and rounded with a faint British affectation.

The Variety Club members were transfixed by his determination to find a smart drug that would kill all of the leukemic cells in a child the way penicillin killed bacteria such as pneumococci and streptococci—without harming the child. Farber wanted to create a clinic for children receiving aminopterin, methotrexate, and other drugs that would surely be developed. His day hospital would have medical specialties, highly trained nurses and pharmacists, social service experts, play therapists, and teachers available to serve children and their parents during treatments with what came to be known as cancer chemotherapy. Above the day hospital would be basic research laboratories in which ever better drugs would be discovered. The entire building would be a cancer center for children, a completely new concept in medicine. If the Variety Club members would support him, they would not be disappointed.

The club members, hunched in their chairs in Farber's cramped office, could not take their eyes off him. His mellifluous, vaguely British voice and carefully chosen words projected complete commitment. The members were mesmerized. They decided to back Sidney Farber and follow him wherever he took them.

With their assistance a new cancer center for children—the day hospital and gleaming research laboratories—rose on a piece of land donated by Children's Hospital. The club members raised the construction money by using their businesses as sources of charitable contributions. They created and exhibited a short film about children with cancer and about the promise of new and effective treatment with antimetabolites. The film was followed by an interruption of the regular movie program during which coin cans were passed like a church collection plate through the captive and somewhat grumbling audience. The cans produced a small but steady stream of support.

Then they had a brainstorm. Television was in its infancy. Ralph Edwards was in the midst of hosting the new medium's most popular program, *Truth or Consequences*. The club members persuaded Edwards to broadcast a special program nationally from Children's Hospital. The program would feature a child with cancer. The patient chosen for the broadcast was a teenager who had undergone surgical removal of a bowel tumor that turned out to be a malignant collection of lymphocytes called a lymphoma. At the time, in 1948, 90 percent of such children died of widespread lymphoblastic lymphoma/leukemia after the operation because the disease had usually already spread to the blood and lymph nodes by the time it was detected. In the end, it became indistinguishable from leukemia. This patient was the first to receive aminopterin after surgery to try to prevent recurrence.

Farber was delighted that his interest in childhood cancer and leukemia/lymphoma in particular was to receive national recognition, but he was anxious to protect the boy's privacy. He was adamant about patient privacy. He regularly covered the faces and genitals of patients during autopsies to protect their dignity and privacy even after death. He refused to allow this patient's real name to be used in the broadcast.

"We'll call him Jimmy," he decided. "Jimmy will be the name for any young boy with cancer."

The television broadcast was a huge success. "Jimmy" came across as a wonderfully courageous young person who was looking death in the eye. Edwards was his usual ebullient self, oozing humor and charm. And as a complete surprise for "Jimmy," members of the then-great Boston Braves baseball team came into the hospital room during the broadcast to present him with a signed baseball bat and a Braves uniform made to fit him. The network producers were ecstatic. The show had everything that television requires: a sick kid who faces a fatal illness with calm and humor, valiant doctors trying to save his life, generous donors who want to raise money to ease distress, plenty of pathos, and celebrity ball players thrown in. It was a brilliant stroke.

This intersection of entertainment and humanitarianism gave birth to the Jimmy Fund, a charity that still appeals to everyone in New England. And in 1953, the Jimmy Fund Building, the new cancer center for children, was ready for occupancy. The Braves left Boston for Milwaukee and then Atlanta, but Tom Yawkey and the Boston Red Sox took over. Walt Disney contributed hand-drawn murals from Pinocchio and Mickey Mouse that have remained on the clinic walls ever since, despite changes in location and remodeling. One of them is autographed by Ted Williams, a tireless supporter of the Jimmy Fund during his playing days.

The Jimmy Fund has a simple message: make your gift, large or small, and cure a kid with cancer now and in the future. The late Cardinal Richard Spellman once called the Jimmy Fund "the little guy's charity," meaning that people in ordinary walks of life can participate and do good. To this day, runners gasp through marathons; cyclists pedal for days until their saddle sores force them to dismount or their muscles collapse; golfers play endless tournaments; police chiefs march; skaters cut figures; and the Red Sox try in vain (until 2004) to win a World Series, all in support of the Jimmy Fund and what became known as the Jimmy Fund Clinic. Every year the fund is more successful than the previous year, and every year clinic progress redoubles the fund's energy.

A huge event occurred in 1997 when "Jimmy," who had been entirely lost to follow-up and whose actual name was no longer known to anyone in the clinic, suddenly turned up as Einar Gustafson, a sixty-three-year-old interstate truck driver from a settlement of Swedes who made his home in the northern reaches of Maine. His sister, a baseball fan, had written to the clinic to tell whoever might open her letter that she believed her brother must be "Jimmy." She thought so because he still owned the bat and the Braves uniform. He had no trace of cancer.

In truth it is very unlikely that the relatively paltry dose of aminopterin that "Jimmy" received had anything to do with his cure. He had been fortunate enough to develop severe symptoms of bowel obstruction and have surgery when the tumor was still small. He was one of the lucky 10 percent who survived the disease before the advent of antimetabolite therapy. Today, nearly all such patients survive because of multiagent chemotherapy.

"Jimmy," at age sixty-three, became a national celebrity (again), driving his new truck with its Jimmy Fund logo all over the United States. He celebrated his newfound notoriety by sharing a reunion in a jammed and tumultuous Fenway Park with Ted Williams. The two heroes spoke movingly of their commitment to the successful treatment of childhood cancer and the cure of cancer in adults as the massive crowd hung on their every word. Then they both rode together around the ball field in a golf cart to accept the screaming ovation of the worshipping fans.

"Jimmy," like Ted Williams, died of stroke complications a few years later. He still had no trace of cancer.

Though Sidney Farber was completely energized by the ten remissions achieved in the first sixteen children, the fact that they all relapsed within a year made him determined to find better drugs and better dose schedules. Farber insisted on giving each chemotherapy agent on its own. If he wanted to test more than one compound in a child, he administered the drugs sequentially. He thought this technique would prevent relapses and prove less toxic to the kids than administering multiple drugs at the same time.

Buttressed by his spacious clinic, staffed with all of the specialists he needed, and out from under the confines of an excellent but antiquated general children's hospital, Farber was in total control of the scientific and clinical agenda for children's cancer. The Jimmy Fund Clinic rapidly became the world epicenter for treatment and research on children's cancer. Pediatricians who wanted to become leaders in the new field called pediatric oncology sought training at the Jimmy Fund Clinic. Among them was Don Pinkel, who later became the first medical director of the new St. Jude Hospital in Memphis. The St. Jude program was created by a popular television entertainer, Danny Thomas, and supported by a group of devoted Lebanese Americans with much of the Variety Club's zeal. The treatment of children's cancer was to become the leading edge of clinical cancer research.

But there was a seemingly immutable problem. All of the children who received a single drug like methotrexate or aminopterin as anti-metabolite chemotherapy relapsed and could no longer be reinduced into remission with either drug even if doses were raised to levels that badly damaged the gastrointestinal tract and created severe mouth sores. It was evident to most investigators that leukemia cells rapidly became resistant to single agents just as some bacteria become resistant to single antibiotics. It would be twenty years before scientists, led by Stanford graduate student Fred Alt, would come to an understanding of how leu-kemic cells may develop resistance. But in the mid-1950s, some forty-five years before Mario's diagnosis, no one understood the mechanism. Far-ber's view was unchanged. To him, the resistance problem would best be solved by a hunt for new drugs that could be given as single agents in sequence. This, he thought, would prevent the emergence of a refractory population of cells and would be less toxic than any other approach.

Despite Farber's unquestioned stature in the field, not everyone was in agreement with him. Abraham Goldin and Lloyd Law at the National Cancer Institute and Howard Skipper and Frank Schabel at the South-ern Research Institute in Alabama did not share his belief in sequential single-agent therapy. Attracted to the field by Farber's discovery of anti-metabolites, these basic scientists studied leukemia cell lines and rodent leukemia model systems under the influence of chemotherapy and con-cluded that Farber was probably wrong. They proposed a simple but profound explanation for the regular emergence of resistance.

At the very beginning of the leukemic process, well before the leu-kemic cells have multiplied to the point at which the disease is actually recognized, the daughter leukemic cells begin to vary subtly from one another. While most of the cells are sensitive to a given dose or schedule of a chemotherapeutic drug, a few are resistant from the very beginning. After the drug destroys the sensitive leukemic cells, the only remaining villains are the resistant ones. They grow and become the dominant pop-ulation. It is a form of survival of the fittest. If a second drug were to be given sequentially, the same events would occur. The two remaining cell populations would be resistant to one or the other drug and treatment would fail. (Fred Alt would later show that the drugs themselves could cause the leukemic cells to become resistant.)

But all was not lost. If the patient (in their case a rodent with leukemia) received a *combination* of two or three or more effective drugs *simultaneously*, a much better outcome would be predicted because it would be unlikely that any cell in the leukemic population would be or would become simultaneously resistant to all of the drugs. The concept of combination chemotherapy was therefore championed by Goldin and Law and a year or two later by Skipper and Schabel. They showed that chemotherapeutic drugs such as antimetabolites and antibiotics work in a unique way. Each dose kills a given fraction of the leukemic cells or bacteria. For example, a certain dose of an antimetabolite chemotherapeutic drug like methotrexate might kill 90 percent of the leukemic cell population. The next dose might kill 90 percent of the residual population, leaving 1 percent of the original population still intact. In this scenario, a minimum residual population would always persist and would eventually comprise the originally resistant leukemic cell population.

The researchers reasoned that combination chemotherapy demands nearly full doses of multiple drugs given simultaneously to achieve maximum cell kill at every dose. As a corollary, they concluded that the best combination would be one that had the highest fractional kill rate, meaning that a combination with a kill fraction of 90 percent would produce more long-term cures than a combination with a kill fraction of 50 percent. The kill fraction could be readily estimated merely by counting the leukemic cells in the blood after each dose.

These scientists readily understood that the limit of their approach would be reached by the toxicity of the combination. For example, if three or four drugs in combination were particularly damaging to normal bone marrow or intestinal cells, the damage from the combination might be so great as to kill the patient (or in their case the rodent) before the leukemia could be cured. So they proposed that active drugs with different toxicities should be combined. Such a proposal was reasonable because drugs tend to be uniquely handled in the body and find their way into different organs. Some primarily damage the liver, some the lung, some the bone marrow, some the nervous system, and others the gut. If several drugs could be developed that were effective against leukemia cells but have variable organ toxicity, combination chemotherapy would be highly useful.

Farber's view of combination chemotherapy and the conclusions drawn from animal experiments was at best sour. "It's fine for rats and mice," he insisted, "but such treatment would injure children terribly. These are all toxic drugs, and I will never allow such experimentation on my children." He went on with his search for a magic bullet, and in 1960 he found one for treatment of another tumor well recognized in pediatrics but a very rare cause of cancer in the general population. Wilms' tumor of the kidney often relapses following surgery because cancer cells are inadvertently left in the operative field or have already metastasized at the time of surgery. Farber tried dactinomycin (Actinomycin D), a newly synthesized antibiotic that was too toxic for use in infectious diseases, and he clearly demonstrated much longer disease-free survival after the use of this single agent following surgery. In fact, many patients were cured. The experience confirmed his unshakable belief that cancer could be cured by single agents given sequentially and that the task of the national cancer effort was to find more and more drugs.

To hasten the search for more drugs, Farber allied himself with Representative John Fogarty of Rhode Island, Senator Lister Hill of Alabama, and Mary and Albert Lasker, both prominent New York philanthropists. They had a huge influence on Congress and on various occupants of the White House. The National Cancer Institute (NCI) budget rose dramatically, and an entire section of the institute focused on testing the anticancer potential of new drugs coming from all over the world.

Two examples reveal the unexpected value of this huge, expensive, and admittedly inefficient effort. The bark of a western yew tree contains a factor that is active against cancer cells. The activity was purified and is known as paclitaxel (Taxol). This yew tree product has become part of the standard treatment for breast cancer. The drug called cisplatin was discovered in a most unusual way. NCI-funded researchers who were examining the effects of an electric current on bacteria uncovered its anticancer activity. They noticed that the bacteria close to a platinum electrode were killed. Platinum is too toxic, particularly to the kidney, to be used to fight infectious diseases, but the NCI screening program helped to show that it is very effective in cancers of the testis and ovary and in a rare and deadly chest tumor known as mesothelioma, which is often seen in asbestos workers.

Though the drugs discovered by the National Cancer Institute, pharmaceutical companies, and independent investigators who made important discoveries by accident were widely different, they had one activity in common: they all seemed to arrest the growth of cells, most by interfering with DNA. Some do it by blocking metabolic pathways that lead to DNA synthesis, as do aminopterin, methotrexate, and 6-mercaptopurine, a compound discovered in 1951 by George Hitchings and Gertrude Elion of Burroughs Wellcome. The three drugs prevent the synthesis of the building blocks of DNA.

Others that were discovered a decade later, such as cytosine arabinoside (AraC), bromodeoxyuridine, thioguanine, and azacytidine, fool DNA into thinking that they are normal building blocks, but once they are incorporated into DNA, they block its reproduction and arrest DNA synthesis. These drugs also create errors in the DNA that *is* made, thereby unleashing the "sniffing" proteins that launch such cells down the death pathway.

Vincristine, a product of the periwinkle plant, and taxol, the drug derived from the bark of yew trees, attack the specialized cellular proteins that are required to pull the DNA-bearing chromosomes of two dividing cells apart. Adriamycin, an anthracycline-based antibiotic, worms its way into DNA and prevents its replication as well as causes errors that alert the sniffing proteins. Unfortunately, it is particularly toxic to the heart.

Asparaginase is an enzyme that destroys the amino acid asparagine, which is required by leukemic lymphoblasts for their protein synthesis. Asparagine is the component of asparagus protein that makes our urine smell peculiar after we eat that vegetable.

Cyclophosphamide, a cousin of the first anticancer drug called nitrogen mustard (a highly toxic and largely abandoned compound discovered after the lethal gas attacks of World War I), diffusely damages DNA and thereby prevents its required doubling before cell division. Finally, Kendall's cortisone, when given at high doses, drives lymphocytes and lymphoblasts down the death pathway by engaging its receptor in the cell nucleus and triggering death genes.

All of these drugs became available between 1948 and 1975. The effort to find them was, in many ways, the result of Farber's influence on national cancer policy.

In the late 1950s and early 1960s, a few enterprising clinical cancer researchers, armed with slowly increasing panels of drugs, became determined to test combination therapy in children with leukemia. Don Pinkel, a bright young pediatrician in the Jimmy Fund Clinic, was getting restless under the firm direction of Sidney Farber. He wanted to try combination chemotherapy. Pinkel knew that if he truly believed in combination treatment, he would have to move to a new location where he could make his own decisions. He first went to the Roswell Park Cancer Institute in Buffalo. In 1961, when the trustees of St. Jude Hospital asked him to become the first medical director of that fledgling children's cancer hospital, he agreed and quickly initiated studies of combination therapy. These studies were at first discouraging but later proved to be highly successful.

Whether Pinkel or others were happy was immaterial to Farber. In the mid-1950s, he established the Jimmy Fund Clinic as the leading institution for excellent and compassionate multidisciplinary pediatric cancer care in the United States—indeed, in the world. By the end of my internship in medicine at the Peter Bent Brigham Hospital in 1956, Farber's stature was close to deification. He was in complete control of cancer care at Children's Hospital and in the Jimmy Fund Clinic, and he had awesome influence in Washington and on the Bethesda campus of the National Institutes of Health. He remained obdurately convinced that single-agent sequential therapy would eventually work and that more aggressive combination chemotherapy would harm the children to whom he was devoted. But when I completed my internship a decade after his initial experiment with Diamond had been launched and set out for the National Cancer Institute, there were still no long-term survivors of childhood leukemia anywhere in the world.

I arrived on the NIH campus in July 1956 to begin a two-year tour of duty as a clinical associate and newly minted U.S. Public Health Service lieutenant. Peter Bent Brigham, where I had served as an intern, then and now (as the Brigham and Women's Hospital) a leading site of academic medicine in the United States, was, like many urban teaching hospitals of the period, a run-down pavilion-type hospital designed and built in 1914. Patients were cared for on large open wards; a thin curtain between each bed served as the only source of privacy. Groans, coughs, spitting, and other loud, unpleasant noises filled the fetid air. The ventilation was terrible. The wards were freezing in the winter, unless one of the miserably hot radiators wheezed into action and banged all night. The whole hospital was stifling in the summer, except in the air-conditioned operating rooms, where some of us occasionally tried to find some sleep on an unused anesthesia bed. Elevators squeaked and rattled as they crept from floor to floor. We never took them because walking the stairs was much faster. The bathrooms for the medical staff were best described as unspeakable. The patient bathrooms were not much better. Some of the laboratories had been remodeled, but most were decrepit. The high productivity of Brigham medical care and research remained a mystery.

The nursing budget in the old Brigham of the 1950s was minimal. During the day shifts, the staffing was reasonable, but after 11:00 p.m., a student nurse, my sole assistant for the entire night, would support a ward of thirty beds. A roving senior resident who was covering half the medical service, and consequently was difficult to find, supervised me. The night nursing supervisor, who would magically appear like the good fairy in *Pinocchio* whenever we were in trouble, oversaw the student nurse. I grew to love nurses because the night supervisor, her heavy chain of keys at her waist and her starched white dress rustling when she moved, seemed to anticipate troubles that, in my limited experience, were impossible to understand. To this day, I stand when a nurse enters the room, because I still remember those times when I relied on nursing supervisors to give me suggestions that would help my patients get through the long night.

The NIH Clinical Center was a shocking study in contrast. It was a massive multiwinged colonial brick building that oozed modernity, with central air conditioning and heating, polished floors, and every conceivable support system including the finest blood bank I had ever seen. The amphitheater looked like a huge movie theater. Courteous elevator operators whisked us from floor to floor. The cafeteria was bright and clean. Above all, the bed floors were spotless; the rooms were designed for two at the most. There were many single rooms, and there were experienced nurses to staff them. Parallel to the hospital beds were corridors of ultramodern laboratories for the physicians.

The Clinical Center was academic medicine heaven. My assignment there even fulfilled the two-year military obligation that I had as a young physician. This was the interbellum period between the conflicts in Korea and Vietnam. America was re-arming and physicians were needed to care for the troops. A small group of interns and residents were given the opportunity to meet their military service requirements by electing to accept an appointment in the Public Health Service at NIH. The U.S. government adopted this policy because the Clinical Center had barely opened and physicians ready to care for the patients or work in the laboratories were already in short supply.

Referral of patients to the Clinical Center was based on a practical reality. These were the days before extensive availability of health insurance and when academic hospitals were in generally deplorable physical condition. If the staff physicians of the National Cancer Institute wanted to study new treatments, they needed only to advertise in medical journals. Practicing physicians with desperate and often uninsured patients would readily refer them to NCI physicians, who would treat them and continue to manage them without charge if they agreed to become research subjects and have their treatment administered on a research protocol. As a clinical associate, it was my job to assist the full-time staff physicians and find a research project of my own.

In that summer of 1956, two recently recruited NCI physicians with similar names and identical goals had committed themselves to a combination chemotherapy attack on childhood leukemia. Emil Frei (known as Tom) and Emil Freireich (known as Jay) had arrived only a few months before me, but by the time I was assigned to their leukemia service as a clinical associate physician, they had established their approach. Combination chemotherapy was about to get an abrupt infusion of energy.

Frei and Freireich began with two experimental drugs, methotrexate and 6-mercaptopurine. Cortisone-like steroids and ACTH (adrenocorticotropic hormone), a pituitary stimulant of cortisone production, were also widely available, but the two investigators did not initially use them. The Eli Lilly pharmaceutical company was reluctantly producing a new extract of the periwinkle plant called vincristine, which was not very effective on its own, but it had an important advantage. Its major toxicity was against the peripheral nervous system and not the gut or the gastrointestinal tract. Methotrexate and 6-mercaptopurine were damaging to the marrow and the intestinal tract but had little or no effect on the nervous system. It appeared that the drugs might be able to be given at full doses simultaneously. But Frei and Freireich faced a serious problem. Eli Lilly wanted to give up on vincristine because it was not very active alone. The NCI group, backed by higher government officials, persuaded the company to manufacture enough for the impending clinical trials.

While waiting for vincristine, Frei and Freireich began with a combination of the antimetabolites methotrexate and 6-mercaptopurine to which prednisone and vincristine would be added later. The leukemic cell count regularly fell rapidly and the remissions were considerably longer when the two antimetabolites were used together, but just as Farber had predicted, the patients became desperately ill from a combination of pancytopenia and gastrointestinal tract damage. Two huge hazards became obvious to the young clinical associates and nurses who were left to care for the patients. One was overwhelming infection from the normal bacteria on the skin and in the gut caused by depletion of the white cells that ingest and kill bacteria. The mucous membranes in the mouth and the intestines also broke down from drug toxicity. Though large doses of intravenous antibiotics could save some of the patients, the bacteria rapidly became resistant to the available antibiotics and many patients would die in shock from massive sepsis.

The liberal use of methotrexate and 6-mercaptopurine and later prednisone severely damaged the patients' normal lymphocyte population. Lymphocytes are made in the lymph nodes and spleen as well as in the marrow. They are necessary to combat viral and fungal infections, and they make the antibodies that fight bacteria. So if children didn't die of bacterial infection from granulocyte (a white blood cell) depletion, their lack of lymphocytes made them vulnerable to any germ that might have been carried into the air of the hospital through the central heating and cooling systems. One fungus, Aspergillus, is a notorious resident of the dusty ducts of central air. Special filters were designed to block its entrance into hospital rooms and corridors, but before the filters were available, Aspergillus was a terrible menace, as were other fungi that lurked in corners of the hospital ready to pounce on these poor compromised children. We were creating combined immune deficiency in these children, and the results were as devastating as the AIDS epidemic today.

The infections were heartbreaking and terrible to behold. A common nasal passage bacterium called *Staphylococcus aureus* had become resistant to penicillin and then to every antibiotic including the combination of erythromycin and chloramphenicol (Chloromycetin) on which we had relied. I remember being called to the bedside of a child with leukemia who had no granulocytes following the combination of 6-mercaptopurine and methotrexate. His fever had spiked to 103, and he had chills. I knew he must have bacteria in his blood, probably staphylococci. He was already on intravenous infusions of all the antibiotics we had available, but I could see red spots appearing on his skin every few minutes. I was sure that the spots were due to clumps of bacteria that had entered a skin blood vessel and started up a local reaction of capillaries. He was dead of shock in a few hours. In another case, I watched a boy with a high fever suddenly become terribly short of breath and observed that his chest was moving like a bellows with each heartbeat. I listened to his heart with my stethoscope and heard a loud whooshing sound between each beat. I realized to my horror that the staphylococci in his blood had lodged on his aortic valve. The bacteria had suddenly eaten through the valve and destroyed it. Every stroke of blood that was ejected from the ventricle fell back uselessly into the chamber. He went into shock and died. One case after another ended in infectious disaster.

The second serious threat was bleeding. The bone marrow produces red cells that carry oxygen, granulocytes that fight infection, and platelets that initiate blood clotting. It is easy to replace red cells with transfusions, but at the time there was no way to transfuse either granulocytes (which live for only a few hours in the blood) or platelets, which live for a week or more but could not be isolated from the blood of donors. The therapeutic plan that Frei and Freireich had developed was based on the understanding that the patient would begin the course of chemotherapy with full doses of methotrexate and 6-mercaptopurine to kill all the leukemia cells. The drugs were damaging to the bone marrow. But they reasoned that once the leukemic cells were dead, the marrow would recover from the drugs and normal blood cell production would resume. That was how mice behaved. But what about human patients?

The answer was not encouraging. The lack of granulocytes and the toxic effects of the drugs on the gastrointestinal tract often caused large ulcers to occur in the mouth and the intestines. The lack of platelets created a constant oozing of blood from these ulcers, and the blood provided a wonderful nesting and growth environment for the bacteria. More hideous infection was the result. Some of the children poured out blood in their stools and in their urine. The pain of the open ulcers in their mouths was terrible, and swabbing them with analgesics made them bleed. Their breath stank from the decaying blood that pooled in their mouths, which they swallowed and vomited. They couldn't eat or drink and had to be fed intravenously. When their temperatures rose, they would bleed into their eyes and out their noses and finally into their brains, and then they were mercifully dead.

For me, this was a nightmare. Sidney Farber seemed to be right. Combination chemotherapy might work for mice, but it was brutal for patients. This wasn't research. It was an execution. I was appalled by what I saw and vowed to find other ways to contribute to medicine. Though I admired them, I thought Frei and Freireich had no idea of the impact of their protocols.

I had a scheduled conference with Gordon Zubrod, the chief of the Medical Service, who had brought Frei and Freireich to NCI and given me my appointment as well. I wanted to talk to him about my own research plans. The late Gordon Zubrod was a gentle, kind, and avuncular man with a charming smile, a soft voice, and a determination to defeat cancer. It was impossible to accuse him of any failure to put patient safety and comfort before science. He began our meeting with a penetrating observation.

"You've had a tough month on the service, David. You haven't seen a single success, and the complications have been very bad. I'm afraid we all endure intervals like this in clinical research. Weeks can go by without any success, and then you may observe a string of much better cases. You've seen nothing but trouble. It reminds me of what happened to Sidney Farber."

"I'm not sure what you mean, Dr. Zubrod. What happened to Sidney Farber?" I asked.

"Oh, coming from Boston, I was sure you knew about it," Zubrod said. "You remember that Sidney and Lou Diamond published their famous paper that claimed that ten of sixteen children with leukemia went into rather long remissions on aminopterin and methotrexate. Well, when Joe Burchenal tried the same drugs on a group of children he treated at Memorial Sloan–Kettering in New York, not one went into remission. For a while, Joe thought the whole thing wasn't true. But since then, other groups have confirmed what Farber and Diamond have claimed. We are going to build a large effort in biostatistics here to help us to understand the variations. We will analyze our results sensibly, and we will confirm whether patients actually go into remission by doing bone marrow exams instead of relying on blood counts. We have a lot of work to do."

He regarded me for a moment. "Before you make up your mind about your own projects for next year, I want you to talk to Tom Frei about the leukemia project. I just want you to consider working on that project and then come back and discuss your future with me."

The next day, I had a long talk with Tom, a tall, thin, bespectacled man who had an encyclopedic knowledge of experimental as well as clinical chemotherapy. I was impressed by him then and remain so today. He listened to me sympathetically and confessed to me that my anxiety about the program was shared both inside and outside the NCI. When I talked to him almost fifty years later, he recalled our discussion.

"David, believe me, you were not the only physician who didn't like what we were doing. We were heavily criticized by nearly everyone— from young trainees like you to very senior and highly influential professors of pediatrics and medicine. I think Gordon Zubrod offered our defense best at a conference at which we were roundly criticized for all of this effort. We were told that it was immoral to experiment on patients who were going to die anyway. At that conference, Gordon said, 'Cure, of course, is our ultimate goal. But we do not expect to make it in one jump. We are going to face each obstacle as it comes: dose escalation, platelet transfusions, combination chemotherapy, central nervous system problems, et cetera.' And we did, and we made it. The first of our publications was in 1960, in which we stated that cure is possible given some of the postulates we have made and some of the results we had. But we certainly had nó cures at the time we wrote that first paper—that encompassed the period when you were with us. The point is that we gradually came to realize that we would have to move from obstacle to obstacle, one step at a time, to manage a disease that we thought could be curable—and turned out to be. Those early experiments taught us the cardinal rule for any cancer. You have to treat hard enough right away to destroy all detectable evidence of tumor. That doesn't guarantee success, but it is a mandatory first step."

I vividly remember that day in 1956. Tom pulled out a sheaf of graphs. "David, here are the results of all the patients we have treated so far with the methotrexate and 6-mercaptopurine protocol. I want you to notice several things. First, over fifty percent of the patients went into a complete bone marrow remission. That's a huge achievement. Second, the rate of decline of the leukemic cell count was very fast in most of them. That says that we were achieving a high rate of cell kill. Now third, let's look at the time between achieving remission and the first sign of relapse. It's much longer than what Farber saw when he used a single agent. We are doing far better with the combination. It's true that we have some bad complications from infection and bleeding, and we have to improve our support systems with platelet and maybe granulocyte transfusions. That will be important. We have to reduce the bleeding and infectious complications. We also need more drugs, and we will soon have vincristine to add to the combination.

"But there is another problem that we are going to have to face. I suspect that some of the leukemic cells are hiding somewhere in the body out of reach of the chemotherapy. If that is the case, we are not going to cure patients even if we get longer remissions. We have to find out about that problem if we are to be successful. We are not going to give up on this."

I was deeply impressed by Tom's sincerity and his approach to the problem. But I knew I didn't have the stomach for this kind of research. Despite the experimental work that seemed to support the effort, the concoctions of drugs were just empirical. Frei and Freireich were simply taking drugs that were available and adding them together in combinations. If one combination didn't work, they would try another. The possible combinations, doses, and schedules of four or five drugs were infinite. Researchers could work for years on finding the right combination of drugs and schedules. I just didn't want to do empirical research, even though the goal was so important. And I had terrible trouble watching the poor patients relapse and suffer from the consequences of pancytopenia and immune depression.

I returned to Zubrod and told him that I wanted to work on a more biochemical problem in patients—something that I could do in the laboratory rather than carrying out cancer clinical trials. He readily agreed and made arrangements for me to work during my second year in a more fundamental research laboratory. But I still had several more months of service caring for patients on experimental protocols before I could turn to the laboratory-based efforts that I would pursue in my second year. In those months, I saw other examples of the potential role of chemotherapy in cancer, one of which was truly amazing.

Choriocarcinoma is a very rare but lethal complication of pregnancy. The cancer cells derive from the placenta and lodge in the inner lining of the uterus, where they begin to grow. The patient notices the disease when she begins to have continuous vaginal bleeding well after the birth of her child. By that time, the disease may already have metastasized to the lungs, and a chest X-ray will reveal massive round lesions in both lung fields. Such a situation is rapidly fatal.

M. C. Li, a junior investigator with a laboratory in the endocrine branch of NCI that was directed by Roy Hertz, somehow had the idea that high doses of methotrexate might work in choriocarcinoma. The cells seem to be multiplying very fast and should be inhibited or killed by an antimetabolite that blocks the folic acid pathway, since cell division demands folic acid. Li was a notoriously difficult but highly intelligent man who flew in the face of conventional thought. He could measure a hormone called choriogonadotropic hormone, which was made by the cancer cells and excreted in the urine. The hormone levels correlated with disease activity. Li's use of the hormone was the first known example of a biochemical marker for cancer that had been devised up to that time.

Li decided that conventional doses of methotrexate would not work and embarked on a high-dose protocol that often caused a lot of mouth sores, intestinal tract problems, and blood count depression, but this protocol did not cause severe pancytopenia. To our amazement, the chest lesions in many of the patients melted away. But Li did not stop treatment. He persisted until all traces of the hormone disappeared from the urine, and he even continued for weeks after that. Many of us could not understand his reasoning, and he was so uncommunicative that it was difficult to keep up with him in any case.

Communication skills notwithstanding, Li cured some of those patients. It was the first example of the use of a single agent to cure a solid tumor—a landmark discovery for which he initially got very little credit. When Li tried to present his discovery to meetings of highly distinguished medical societies such as the American Society of Clinical Investigation, he was turned down. As one of my Harvard Medical School classmates, John Laszlo, wrote in his book, *The Cure of Childhood*

*Leukemia in the Age of Miracles*, academic medicine has its own snob clubs. In those days, cancer clinical researchers were unwelcome in many circles because the field was seen as a "try one–try another" empirical guessing game for which there was no scientific basis. Only laboratory-based science was acceptable. (Li received a Lasker Prize in 1972.)

I had trouble in some of my interactions with Li, but the disappearance of those chest lesions remained in my mind. Chemotherapy had a future, I was certain of it; but its application in leukemia seemed far away. As for the rest of the cancers that I saw, there seemed to be little or no progress. Metastatic breast cancer, the wildly malignant sarcomas of the bone and cartilage or the outer layers of the gut, and hormone-resistant prostate cancer were all beyond the reach of the oncologists of the 1950s. But I did not realize that a major change was on the way in leukemia and that the progress in those malignancies would spark a revolution in cancer management.

At NCI, the investigations of childhood leukemia continued. The four-drug combination of vincristine, amethopterin (methotrexate), 6-mercaptopurine, and prednisone now had an acronym known as VAMP. Inexorably, the rate of cell kill increased, the incidence of achievement of first remission improved, and the length of time between the first remission and relapse was progressively extended. The terrible toxicity that I observed was reduced with improved antibiotics, newly developed platelet transfusions, and even granulocyte transfusions. And of seventeen patients, three were actually cured: the first three patients to be cured of leukemia. Though the vast majority of the patients eventually relapsed, the longer life span of the patients provided important clinical clues that finally explained many of the relapses.

A few boys with leukemia developed swollen testicles during the courses of chemotherapy, and biopsy would reveal leukemic cells in the testes. Clearly the drugs struggled to gain access to the testis, which provided a sanctuary for leukemic cells. Far more common were cases of what appeared to be spinal meningitis that occurred during treatment and turned out to be due to leukemic cell infiltration of the lining of the brain and spinal cord.

Frei and Freireich treated the cases of leukemic meningitis with injections of methotrexate into the spinal fluid via a lumbar puncture. In several cases, the cells disappeared. That gave them an important idea.

Suppose, they mused, that all of the patients actually have leukemic cells in their spinal fluid just lurking there. When given by mouth or vein, the drugs penetrate the spinal fluid very poorly because a biologic barrier that is designed to protect the brain prevents the drug from entering the brain and the spinal cord where the leukemic cells are hiding. The leukemic cells in that fluid will be ready to reemerge into the blood to start the disease all over again unless additional doses of the drug are injected directly into the spinal fluid to kill the cells that are hiding there.

The idea of central nervous system *prophylactic* chemotherapy with methotrexate became a central theme of the NCI team's effort, and it provided the first big steps toward success. Don Pinkel, then at St. Jude Hospital, used external radiation to the brain and the spinal cord together with VAMP and achieved results similar to those of the NCI team. By the mid- to late 1960s, the cure rate of childhood lymphoblastic leukemia with combination chemotherapy and central nervous system prophylaxis had increased to a bit more than 30 percent. The fact that the central nervous system may be a sanctuary for cancer cells is now appreciated by adult oncologists, as they are increasingly seeing patients with breast or lung cancer, who seem to be disease-free in the rest of the body, relapse in the brain. Though childhood leukemia is a rare disease, it has pointed the way to effective treatment of the common adult cancers.

Tom Frei was eighty years old in 2005 and physically limited by Parkinson's disease. His career has been wonderfully distinguished. He rose in the ranks at NCI to become chief of the medicine branch, then head of the Department of Developmental Therapeutics at M.D. Anderson Cancer Center in Houston, and in 1974 he became president of the Dana-Farber Cancer Institute following the death of Sidney Farber. Justifiably, Frei, Freireich, and Pinkel are recipients of some of the highest awards in medical research, among them the coveted General Motors Prize and the Lasker Award. But Frei readily admits that the early days of his work at NCI were hard on the patients and on the staff.

In the early 1970s, now chief of Hematology at Children's Hospital and in charge of referring children with leukemia to the Jimmy Fund Clinic, I had to tell Dr. Farber that I could no longer refer patients to him if he would not adopt the successful combination chemotherapy program that the NCI and St. Jude investigators had established.

As far as I could tell, Farber never went home. The lights in his office on the top floor of the Jimmy Fund Clinic burned well into the night. I knew from previous visits that he had a complete washroom and shower in the office, and there was a comfortable sofa on which he could find an hour or two of sleep. Otherwise, he worked on a policy issue, an effort to raise funds, or a promising approach to a new cancer drug.

I dreaded this particular appointment with him. I had had previous encounters in which I had asked him to consider combination therapy. His face had reddened and he had waved me off abruptly each time.

On the way to the Jimmy Fund Clinic, I happened to see Dr. William Berenberg, the favorite pediatrician at Children's Hospital and a confidant of Dr. Farber.

"Look out for the match trick," called Berenberg.

"What's the match trick?" I asked.

"You'll see," Berenberg answered.

I entered the Jimmy Fund Clinic and apprehensively took the elevator to the eighth floor. By the time I reached Farber's office, my mouth was dry and my heart rate elevated. I sat in the waiting room for what seemed to be hours. Then with a rustling sound, the tall door opened and Farber stood in the doorway clad in his perfect white coat. Mine looked wrinkled, and I noted that the cuffs were a bit dirty as I entered that top-floor office and prepared to begin what would become my final meeting with him.

He placed me in a somewhat unaccommodating chair at the corner of his rich walnut desk. Standing alone in front of me on the corner of the beautifully finished wood surface was a gray stone bird, its sharp beak extended upward and its red eye staring at me. Above the bird's aggressive head was Dr. Farber's. His once black hair and mustache had become very gray and his face was pale. I tried not to stare back and began my litany about the need to adopt combination therapy.

He interrupted me before I had gotten out more than a sentence or two.

"Dr. Nathan, I know very well how you feel about combination therapy, but thankfully you are not responsible for the care of these children, and you are not in a position to inflict this punishment on them. I am responsible, and I will simply not adopt a form of therapy that injures so many in an effort to rescue a few. There's no point in a further argument. You have your views and you are entitled to them, but I have the responsibility, and as long as I have it, we will not do what you suggest."

I realized that the situation was hopeless and informed him as grace-fully as I could that I would no longer refer patients from Children's Hospital to him or to the Jimmy Fund Clinic unless he guaranteed a change in the therapy. At that point, Farber's face turned bright red and his hands began to tremble. I became very concerned because I knew he had a history of coronary disease and hypertension. I thought he might have a stroke in front of me. But he regained his composure and slowly opened the drawer of his desk to remove a wooden match. He held up the match between the thumb and middle finger of his left hand, snapped it in half, and threw the pieces on the desk in front of me.

"I'll break you like that," he said in a near whisper of barely con-trolled rage.

I stared at the match fragments and made a terrible error. "My God," I whispered audibly. "That's the match trick."

With that, Farber simply lost it. He stood at the desk, his fists on the surface as he hunched over them, and shouted at me to get out of the office and never come back. I never saw him again. That was a much bigger loss for me than for him. He died in his office shortly after that terrible interview while working far into the night on a strategy for cur-ing cancer in children. Here was a truly great clinical scientist who made a huge contribution to cancer research, but he could not engage in the approaches that his own science had initiated. He had, in effect, opened a new pathway that he himself could not follow. But recognizing that his health was failing, he made the decision in 1973 to bring Tom Frei, one of combination therapy's great advocates, to Dana-Farber to become the physician in chief. The understanding was that Tom would take over when Farber relinquished authority. With that decision, Farber admit-ted to himself that combination therapy was the way to go. He simply could not let it happen on his own watch. The risks of hurting a child very badly were more than he could bear.

And there matters stood until the next phase began. In 1974, when Sidney Farber died, Tom Frei became president of Dana-Farber. Tom invited me to form a newly combined Children's Hospital/Dana-Farber Cancer Institute pediatric hematology and oncology program. I asked a young trainee, Stephen Sallan, to be the clinical director of the new pro-gram and work closely with Tom to establish therapeutic approaches featuring combination chemotherapy.

Sallan is a very tall man with big hands and feet and a large disposition. He is quite nearsighted, so he stays close to people when he talks, and he has a soothing calmness about him. He came to the Jimmy Fund Clinic and the oncology program at Dana-Farber and Children's Hospital after his training in pediatrics, a tour of duty in the submarine service of the navy, and a year of child psychiatry. To this day, I do not know how Steve was able to manipulate his very tall body through the rabbit warren of a submarine, but he could readily ingratiate himself into the loyalties of his colleagues and the trust of the patients and their families.

In 1974, the VAMP protocol, coupled with treatment of the central nervous system, was producing a cure rate in ALL children of less than 40 percent. Steve and Tom set out to improve those results. The key decision that helped significantly was to add two more drugs to the VAMP regimen. These were the enzyme asparaginase (an old-timer that rids the body of the amino acid asparagine and had fallen largely out of favor) and Adriamycin, a fairly recently isolated antibiotic that is very toxic to many tumor cells (and normal cells) because it damages DNA. Adriamycin and its closely related analogue, daunomycin, are particularly toxic to heart muscle and must be used with great care, and asparaginase damages the pancreas.

Steve and Tom knew that the six-drug protocol (which was used to induce Mario into remission) and radiation to the brain would be toxic and that some children would be injured, but they forged ahead because they were determined to increase the cure rate. Their persistence was rewarded. Over the course of the next twenty years, Steve and several collaborating pediatric oncology programs raised the cure rate from less than 40 percent to more than 80 percent. Steve explained the rationale this way:

"In the absence of more specific treatment like smart drugs that would kill a leukemic cell specifically, the original concept of Frei and Freireich was to deliver known antileukemic drugs that had different mechanisms of leukemia cell killing at their maximal tolerated doses. By giving them together, they hoped to overcome resistance mechanisms and endure acceptable toxicity. These are all principles to which we still adhere today. But our team recognized that there was a lot of individual variation in dose tolerance, and for the first time in the mid-1970s, we wrote guidelines for the individual patient to have doses adjusted downward or upward based on what we considered safe blood cell counts. I realize that we were functioning empirically, but it was the best we could do to predict dangerous toxicity.

"Then we had to decide how long to treat the patients. The duration of treatment in the early 1970s was thirty months or two years after entering complete remission. Half of the patients who had stopped treatment at that point stayed in remission. But, of course, 50 percent of children who completed treatment would go on to relapse. To deal with that in the late 1970s and early 1980s, we intensified treatment in patients at higher risk of relapse (such as those with T-cell ALL). More intensive treatment meant that after remission was induced, we would continue treatment for two years with high doses of methotrexate, coupled with as much asparaginase as could be tolerated. One of the really major accomplishments in our own program was to show that prolonged depletion of the amino acid asparagine by asparaginase could make a huge difference in leukemia-free long-term survival.

"After we intensified treatment, we found that the majority of children had fewer relapses during therapy and had fewer relapses after cessation of treatment as well. This suggested that we were not merely suppressing the disease only to have it reappear after cessation, but in fact we were eradicating more leukemia. There was also a decrease in the number of off-therapy relapses and a big decrease in the incidence of testicular leukemia. When we started to become successful in our treatments in the early 1970s and into the early 1980s, boys often had testicular relapse as their first sign of disease. By the 1990s, that phenomenon almost disappeared, and it is less than 1 percent today.

"Perhaps the most important lesson I've learned from all of this is that there is a real struggle in this field between those who insist on greater efficacy and those who demand less toxicity; this struggle has been a subtext of the whole pediatric oncology movement.

"We are now curing over 80 percent of these children. The next task is to cure the remaining 15 percent, of which Mario is an unfortunate member. To conquer their cancers, we will need smart drugs that target the precise genetic pathways that drive leukemia in those patients. Scott's work on Mario's case will help us get there."

It is important to emphasize that Sallan's protocols and those of like-minded colleagues in Europe and the United States did cause considerable toxicity. A small but real percentage of the children who were cured of leukemia suffered from drug- or radiation-induced heart disease, learning disabilities, pancreas insufficiency, liver disease, and other difficulties. But they are alive, and the physicians who treated them had their survival as their primary goal. What is needed is a reliable method of sorting those patients who need more intensive chemotherapy from those who do not.

The relatively new science called molecular cytogenetics is helping Sallan and his colleagues sort the chemotherapy-resistant and the sensitive childhood leukemias from one another. In ordinary cytogenetics, a technician looks at a preparation of leukemia cell chromosomes and finds a diagnostic chromosome translocation if it is there. But some translocations are so small that they elude the eye of even a skilled technician. In such cases, the abnormally fused chromosomes and the fused genes that ensue can be detected by means of probes made of DNA itself. This is called molecular cytogenetics. For example, in contrast to the relatively rare MLL translocation, which connotes a very poor prognosis, a common translocation involving two other genes called TEL and AML1 connotes an excellent prognosis. Molecular cytogenetics has made those important distinctions possible.

DNA probes and molecular cytogenetics have also been utilized to define the risk of relapse in individual patients. In 2005, Sallan, Silverman, and their colleague, John Gribben, completed a very important analysis of children treated for ALL. They studied the marrows of 308 patients with the common B-cell type of ALL who had undergone induction of visually apparent complete remission with combination chemotherapy. They examined those marrows with highly sensitive DNA probes to detect invisible leukemia cells, and they followed the patients for five years. They found that only 3 percent of patients who had no DNA probe–detectable leukemic cells after induction ever relapsed. In contrast, 43 percent of those who had DNA probe–detectable leukemic cells after remission induction ultimately relapsed. Clearly the second group (which certainly includes the unfortunate children with MLL leukemia) requires much more intensive and sustained therapy than the first group.

Given the prognostic importance of the MLL translocation in childhood leukemia, the final decision on Mario's treatment would await the molecular cytogenetic analysis of his leukemic DNA to determine whether the MLL gene was involved. But I am getting ahead of the story about Mario's diagnosis and treatment.

# CHAPTER FOUR

# The Final Treatment Plan for Mario

Doctors finally brought an exhausted Flavia some good news. Mario's life-threatening leukemic cell count had declined in response to the blood transfusion and two low doses of the chemo agent Adriamycin. After the boy was transferred back to the oncology unit, Scott Armstrong again explained to the parents that Mario would have to stay in the hospital for the next month during the first intense phases of chemotherapy. The cancer-fighting medicines would drive his normal white cell count to very low levels and make him extremely vulnerable to infection. He might not survive such an infection were he forced to use precious time traveling from home to the emergency ward. Dark circles surrounded Flavia's eyes as she looked around Mario's room and realized that it would be home for both of them.

Scott's next job was to determine with certainty that Mario had MLL leukemia. If he did, he would need a second month of intense chemotherapy and thus an additional month in the hospital.

Scott received the diagnostic answer from the molecular cytogeneticists two weeks after Mario began his difficult one-month therapy program. The boy had MLL leukemia. Scott scheduled another meeting with the parents in the "bad news room." Mario's illness had already exacted a severe toll on the family. Flavia was clearly worn out. She had not left her son's room other than to go to the cafeteria to eat listlessly. She had slept poorly in her cot next to his bed and had been awakened by the nurses at night when they turned on the lights to take his pulse, blood pressure, and temperature. Walter, who had been living at home, was more composed, but he was suffering an enormous psychological burden, desperately trying to achieve a sense of control over the situation.

Flavia and Walter remember every grim detail of that conference. Walter remembers the meeting as though it happened yesterday. Scott "dropped the bomb" there, he says, and "we died a little bit again." Scott told the parents the chances for curing Mario "weren't as good as we had hoped for," perhaps on the order of fifty-fifty.

To deal emotionally with the first round of treatment, the parents had decided that Mario's case wasn't that dangerous. They convinced themselves that the leukemia was the good kind, Walter explained, and that given Mario's response, his body would defeat the cancer. The parents figured they were "beating all of the odds," he recalled. "We even went to the point of saying, 'This is good, this looks great.' But when Scott told us differently, it was as though somebody pulled the rug from right underneath us. It really hit us."

Still, they held tight to a bit of the rug. Over time, Walter and Flavia began to understand Scott's research and the reasons for his treatment approach. "I remember telling Flavia that having Scott with us was like sending your letter to Santa and getting what you asked for," Walter remembered. "Thank God, we had Scott."

"We had the choice of who we wanted to work with," Flavia said. "Scott always had that very down-to-earth way. Every time I talked to him, I would ask him, how sure are you of that? And he would say, 'As sure as I look.' He never gave me more hope or less hope. He was always very honest. Many times, I would say, do you think this or that? He would say, 'I wish I could tell you that. I wish I could tell you that it's going to be fine, . . . but we don't know how it's going to work.'"

Walter added, "We grilled him. We asked him every question we could think of and some we cannot even remember. And he answered us truthfully and calmly. We grew to love him."

Scott explained that the evidence was now crystal clear. Mario had MLL. Until only a decade before Mario's admission, MLL had been considered uniformly fatal. Though the outlook was certainly less favorable than for standard ALL, there had been major progress in fighting MLL over those ten years. Lew Silverman, who was experienced in delivering such news, coached Scott in what to say:

"The outlook for childhood leukemia has improved significantly over the last couple of decades and we have made great strides, but you know that not all childhood leukemia is the same. Leukemia, when it develops in very young children like Mario, seems to be more resistant to the drugs that we have available. Children between the ages of four and twelve respond better to the treatment. The odds are not as good for the very young child or for the child older than twelve." Lew continued, "We were doing very poorly with the infants until the late 1980s. In 1987, for example, we were able to control the leukemia in infants for a while, but in the vast majority of cases, particularly those with Mario's MLL leukemia, the leukemia would come back."

At that time, the chances of cure were very low. Nationally, the estimated long-term survival was below 10 percent. Lew had advised Scott not to volunteer such bad news in the initial discussion of the overall plan, and he didn't. But both Lew and Scott realized that Flavia and Walter would then ask how long Mario might live. What's more, they would ask that question of everyone on the medical team, in one way or another. There had to be a uniform response.

Lew advised Scott to respond along these lines:

"That is always a very hard question to answer, and it is impossible to know with any child what is going to happen. It is true that infant leukemia tends to come back fairly early after we treat it, so it is possible that the leukemia will return within the first two years of treatment. But we have intensified the treatment recently; we have added a second month, using some agents that we do not normally use for older kids with ALL. One of these drugs is cytarabine (AraC). We have excellent evidence that it is improving the outlook for babies. And we have added two extra injections of a third compound that has been used by the team for a few years. It is too early to know how successful this approach will be, but we are already seeing much better results, and that makes me feel more hopeful that we may be able to cure Mario."

Lew and Scott had excellent reasons to believe that such a statement would be truthful and supportable. But because they were working with an orphan disease—one that affects a very small number of people—they couldn't offer statistically useful findings. As described in chapter 3, they had achieved encouraging results after adopting a second month of intensive treatment with AraC in twenty-three leukemic infants, eleven of whom had MLL. Fifty percent of those infants had survived disease-free. At the time of Mario's admission in 1999, an international study had just begun with far more patients to determine whether the preliminary results would be confirmed. There were no data available from the international study when Mario was admitted, but the preliminary study had implied that the new therapy could achieve nearly 50 percent long-term survival in all babies with ALL and suggested that such an improved survival could be achieved in babies with leukemia and proven translocations involving MLL. That was an important finding, and it influenced Scott to be cautiously optimistic in his discussion with Walter and Flavia.

There was other information that had just entered the circle of leukemia specialists. Just before Mario's admission, a group of pediatric oncologists in Germany had confirmed the preliminary findings of Sallan and Silverman with an important additional finding. They reported that babies also did very well after a month of AraC, following a one-week course of a steroid called prednisone.

Further confirmation had come from Dutch pediatric oncologists who showed that leukemic lymphoblasts from babies with MLL seemed more sensitive to AraC than to other drugs. There was growing international agreement that AraC and high-dose early prednisone might play important roles in defeating infant leukemia. The international treatment plan, used in the United States, Germany, Holland, and Canada, begins with prednisone and continues with AraC and frequent doses of methotrexate. These encouraging results became available in 2004, well after Mario had completed his entire course of treatment.

Scott explained the background to Flavia and Walter as simply and directly as he could. His bottom line was this recommendation: After Mario completed the first month of induction treatment in the hospital, he could go home for two or three days, then return to the hospital for a second month. During that time, he would receive five chemotherapy drugs including AraC. After his bone marrow recovered from this onslaught, Mario would receive a course of radiation to his brain and chemotherapy injections into his spinal fluid as well as more chemotherapy, at a total dose that had been chosen for patients with a high risk of relapse.

After that huge amount of treatment, Mario could go home, but he would still receive chemotherapy as an outpatient in the Jimmy Fund Clinic. He would receive four of the drugs every three weeks and two others every four months. Adriamycin would be stopped at a certain point to avoid damage to the heart. In all, the chemical pummeling would end two years after he had entered complete remission.

While Flavia and Walter tried to absorb all that information, Scott began another discussion that described a different approach: bone marrow transplantation. Following achievement of complete remission by chemotherapy, this technique would involve giving Mario a very large dose of chemotherapy delieverd over four days and radiating his entire body. He would then receive an infusion of bone marrow cells from a donor who matched his immunological features as closely as possible.

But the treatment is a perfect example of a medical double-edged sword. The huge blast of chemo-radiation therapy may be terribly toxic to the skin, lungs, gastrointestinal tract, brain, and liver. One or more of these systems might not recover, and they cannot be replaced. Marrow transplant can be associated with severe pulmonary failure or liver failure or both. Marrow-transplanted patients may fail to engraft (a rare complication, particularly in children), and they may have extremely slow recovery of donor T-lymphocytes, a condition known as immunodeficiency. T-lymphocytes are the normal cells that can kill leukemic cells, and they are responsible for the killing of viruses and fungi.

In the period of severe posttransplant immunodeficiency due to T-lymphocyte depletion, Mario might succumb to an overwhelming viral or fungal infection. And even if the donor T-lymphocytes did numerically recover in Mario, they might have little or no antileukemia, antiviral, and antifungal functions; they might "see" Mario's own tissues as foreign and viciously attack them. That unfortunate state of affairs is called graft versus host disease, an illness characterized by severe dermatitis and gastrointestinal and liver dysfunction. Immunosuppressive drugs can ameliorate this disease, but the drugs limit the antileukemic effects of the T-lymphocytes. Therefore, the management and prevention of graft versus host disease provides an excellent example of what some of my British colleagues call "gaining at the circle and losing at the roundabout."

Though marrow transplantation is hazardous and particularly dangerous in infants and very young children with chemoradiotherapy-sensitive nervous systems, it has been successfully performed in older children and adults thousands of times throughout the world largely because of the efforts of E. Donnell Thomas, of Seattle, Washington, who pioneered the field and received a Nobel Prize for his work. Children have also been treated successfully with marrow transplantation for acquired and congenital bone marrow failure. Very young children present a special case because their nervous systems are still developing. A high dose of radiation therapy delivered over a four-day period could seriously undermine the neurological development of an infant.

Despite the hazards, bone marrow transplantation offers two advantages over relying largely on chemotherapy for the treatment of leukemia. The time required for treatment is much shorter, since the treatment is extremely intense. The other benefit is that while the blood cells emanating from the newly transplanted bone marrow stem cells are immunologically compatible, they are not completely so. The slightly incompatible cells might detect and destroy the few leukemic cells that have survived the firestorms of chemotherapy and radiation.

Lew Silverman opposed the idea of a bone marrow transplant for Mario. It would present another huge challenge to Mario's body. Also, Mario did not have a sibling who could donate bone marrow. A brother or a sister has a one in four chance of being a close immunological match, but greater genetic diversity would increase the likelihood of Mario's rejecting the graft or developing graft versus host disease. For this child, the medical team would have to use a worldwide marrow cell registry to search for a suitable donor. That such a donor could be found was a reasonable probability, but the compatibility would not be as great as that from using a sibling.

Lew also felt that Mario's age (nineteen months) posed a special hazard. His brain might not tolerate the very high dose of chemotherapy and radiation that must be used to ensure a successful marrow graft. Furthermore, Lew was of the opinion that MLL leukemia is simply not sensitive enough to the short-term huge dose of chemo-radiation treatment that characterizes the transplant protocol. He advised strongly against the procedure.

But when Scott talked to the professional marrow transplanters at Children's Hospital and Dana-Farber about that last point, he got a somewhat different opinion. Pediatric oncologists from other centers had referred MLL patients to them for transplant, and their results were on average about the same as they achieved in other childhood leukemias.

However, the total number of MLL transplants was too small to draw any firm conclusions.

So the role of marrow transplant in childhood leukemia remains a matter of opinion. It seemed to Scott and to Lew that the risks definitely outweighed the benefits in a case in which a matched unrelated donor was necessary. Scott reported all this to Flavia and Walter, who took the chemotherapy option. They did not want to roll the dice. They opted for the prolonged chemotherapy, hoping that it would edge the leukemia out of Mario in several months rather than bludgeoning it out in a few weeks. The risk of the bludgeoning was simply too high. It is very likely that their choice was largely based on their newfound faith in Scott. Flavia and Walter trusted him and bought a two-year treatment ticket for their son.

# CHAPTER FIVE

# The Risk of Chemotherapy Resistance

When Flavia and Walter agreed to the two-year course of chemotherapy for Mario, they were relying on the hope that Mario's MLL leukemic cells would not become resistant to the potent combinations of drugs that would be visited on him by Scott Armstrong, Lew Silverman, and their colleagues. Mario's parents did not want to contemplate that risk closely; they asked few questions about the development of resistance. But the risk never left Scott's mind as he began the complex protocol he would deliver over the next twenty-four months.

Scott and Lew had only a student's view of cancer chemotherapy resistance. They had never studied the phenomenon in the laboratory and probably were unaware of how mysterious the resistance was to those who had encountered it during the early days of chemotherapy for leukemia in the 1960s.

I had seen chemotherapy resistance develop rapidly in the children I cared for at NCI in the 1950s. At that time, I had no idea how it happened. Somehow cells that appeared to be sensitive to chemotherapeutic agents lost their sensitivity and did not regain it. This mystery was not resolved until Fred Alt, a fledgling graduate student, arrived at Stanford University in 1971. Amazingly, although his field was plant physiology, he solved an important part of the puzzle.

Fortunately, Fred, now one of the leading basic immunologists in the United States, is a close colleague. I recruited him to Children's Hospital when I was chief of pediatrics there. I knew he had cracked much of the mystery of resistance, but I had never had a chance to talk to him about the big discovery he had made thirty years previously. Mario's battle with MLL inspired me to ask him about his approach to the problem during his graduate student days. He had made the discovery in his very first foray into research in mammalian cells. Such a discovery is a rare event in the life of any graduate student, and I looked forward to learning his story.

Fred began with a brief review of his family background and his choice of career. He had always had a deep interest in life science and loved studying general biology when he was growing up. Orphaned by the time he was eleven—his mother died of breast cancer when he was eight and his father of prostate cancer three years later—he became acutely aware of cancer. From that time forward, Fred always wanted to work on a cure.

He attended high school in Johnstown, Pennsylvania, where he lived with his older sister. It so happened that the school had extremely good science and math teachers. "They were unbelievable," Fred recalled. Stimulated by his teachers, Fred took various biology courses in the summer. He went to college at Brandeis University, where he worked in a very good, basic science lab on plant physiology. "Clearly a lot of my interests were not in plant physiology, but it was good science, and when you are doing good science, you can get excited. Who knows? It could end up being relevant," Fred pointed out.

He went on to Stanford in 1971 to pursue a Ph.D. Those were the early days of the burgeoning science of gene regulation, and Alt found that subject far more interesting than plant physiology. He decided to find mentors who could teach him much more about genes and how to study their action in animal cells. During his search, he became fascinated by the work of the late Gordon Tompkins at the University of California in San Francisco. Tomkins studied the development of drug resistance in cultured animal cells. Alt had followed his papers from the time he was an undergraduate. As a graduate student, he also sat in on some dynamic classes taught by Bob Schimke, a young Stanford professor who was also dealing with issues related to drug doses and drug resistance.

Under the influence of those researchers, Alt began to devour papers dealing with the phenomenon of resistance to methotrexate in cancer cells. He learned that the compound inhibits DNA synthesis by jumping onto and blocking the function of an enzyme called DHFR (dihydrofolate reductase; an enzyme is a protein that regulates the rate of biochemical reactions in cells) that is essential for DNA production. Without the DHFR enzyme, cells lose the ability to synthesize DNA and they die.

When given alone, methotrexate eventually becomes useless in the face of leukemic cells; they become resistant to it. Then they return to flood the blood, the marrow, and the vital organs, thereby killing the patient. Tompkins and Schimke did not know how cancer cells become resistant to drugs, so Alt decided to get to the bottom of it. This was his first animal cell research project.

Schimke and Tompkins had set the stage for Alt by carrying out a set of illuminating experiments. They grew mouse cancer cells in a culture dish and added a dose of methotrexate to those cultures. Almost all the cells were killed, but some survived and continued to grow. When a higher dose of methotrexate was added, most of those cells died, but once again, some survived. Eventually, the team could produce cancer cells that resisted massive doses of methotrexate.

Alt decided to find out how the cells accommodated ever-larger doses of methotrexate and what was happening to the genes that control the production of the DHFR enzyme protein. His initial approach was to measure the absolute amount of the DHFR enzyme in the resistant cells. He had to produce an antibody to the enzyme—a task that took months. But Alt did it and found his answer—the amount of enzyme protein was markedly increased in the resistant cells. Cancer cells made increasing amounts of the DHFR enzyme as the dose of methotrexate rose. This is how they resist the drug. Killing all cancer cells with any dose of methotrexate that could be tolerated by patients' normal cells is impossible, he concluded. He knew that the drug causes the DHFR genes to make more DHFR enzyme protein. The next step was to determine how the genes make the extra protein.

Alt's choices were simple in concept but technically difficult. There were two possible explanations for the surprising finding that the DHFR genes in the tumor cells could actually increase their production of DHFR enzyme protein. The first and simplest was that in the presence of methotrexate, the appropriate genes—the DHFR genes—remained intact in their places on the chromosomes but somehow increased their production of the DHFR enzyme. If so, that would mean that the drug must induce a small mutation in one or both copies of the two normal DHFR genes in the cancer cells—so-called point mutations that would cause faster production of the DHFR enzyme from the mutated gene. But that idea did not seem right to Alt. The induction of point mutations—the actual changing of the base sequence of DNA—takes time, and the effect of methotrexate on resistance and increased DHFR enzyme protein production was very rapid. Furthermore, Alt did not have the tools to sequence any gene and find a point mutation.

The second possibility seemed unlikely but possible. Methotrexate might actually damage DNA and the region around the DHFR genes and induce those genes to copy themselves. The larger number of genes would make more DHFR enzyme protein simply because there were more than two copies of the gene in the cells. The number of DHFR genes might be roughly proportional to the dose of methotrexate—the more drug, the more genes, the more enzymes, the more resistance, and the more cancer cell production.

Determining that more genes were produced by exposure to the drug required the development of both a new technology and a change in the accepted dogma of genetics. Almost all scientists at that time thought genes (particularly animal and human genes) were stable structures. After all, an offspring inherits one copy of each gene from each parent. That number does not change. The idea that genes might increase in number by copying themselves was not an accepted notion. And practically, there were no easy ways to measure the number of genes. Today, the experiment Alt needed to answer his questions would take a few hours. But in the early 1970s, measuring a critical component of what we now call the genome, such as the number of copies of a particular gene in a cell, required extremely laborious work.

To make matters more difficult, Alt was under the pressure of time. He had lined up a coveted postdoctoral fellowship with David Baltimore at the Massachusetts Institute of Technology. The project he would pursue upon entering Baltimore's lab in 1977 had nothing to do with DHFR and methotrexate resistance. So Alt started to think about ways to move his DHFR project at Stanford along more swiftly. He was becoming increasingly convinced that methotrexate resistance came about because of growth in the quantity of DHFR genes. The speed with which the cells became resistant when doses of methotrexate were raised and the speed with which they regained sensitivity when doses were lowered convinced him that changes in gene numbers were quite likely. But he still needed to devise an experiment that would prove his point. Science is not about conviction. It is about data.

Then Alt had a fortunate break. He came across some papers on antibiotic resistance in bacteria. In certain bacteria, such resistance comes about when the bacteria acquire viruslike particles that contain a gene that produces an enzyme that destroys the antibiotic. When bacteria are hit with higher doses of the antibiotic, the viruslike particles and the gene they contain increase and the bacteria produce ever more copies of the enzyme. When the drug is removed, the particle numbers go down, as do the numbers of genes and enzymes. Those papers confirmed Alt's growing conviction that he had to find a way to measure the DHFR gene number in cancer cells with and without methotrexate exposure.

"To make that measurement, I knew I would need a radioactive copy of the DHFR gene to use as a probe," Fred explained. The technology had just been established in a laboratory at the University of California, San Francisco. "It occurred to me that it would be very simple to use those genetic techniques to make a probe to find DHFR genes."

As Alt tells the story of his first critically important triumph, a gleam comes into his eyes and his voice becomes animated. Sometimes science resembles a sporting event in which the scientist is pitted against a recalcitrant nature that does not want to give away any points. Alt had to struggle to make the probe, and he had to have an ingenious approach. Thirty years after he worked out his technique, he still finds the memory gratifying. "The first time I tried, it worked unbelievably well," he said.

The measurement with the probe took all night. In the morning, Fred had his answer. Methotrexate resistance is due to the growth of the number of DHFR genes, which in turn come from the drug's presence. The amount of drug in the cells induces resistance to it—a classic case of survival of the fittest. He repeated the experiments successfully and then wrote about them.

Today, that article is a classic in the cancer treatment literature. Alt proved that at least one form of cancer chemotherapy resistance is due to the increased numbers of copies of the gene that makes the protein the target of the drug. The realization that cancer cells could actually take advantage of cancer chemotherapy by multiplying their genes, thereby preventing the toxic action of a drug, was a revelation to cell biologists.

And it was a severe disappointment to cancer chemotherapists. This effect of methotrexate is not limited to the DHFR gene. Many genes are amplified in methotrexate-treated cells. Another of these genes produces a protein that acts like a pump in reverse of the one that forces MLL cells to suck up AraC. This pump is pernicious because it kicks many drugs out of the cell. Just by itself, methotrexate may cause that pump gene to amplify, produce many pumps, and lead to resistance to quite a few drugs. That pump gene, which has been named the multidrug resistance gene, plays havoc with combination chemotherapy. The more closely we look at cancer cells, the more we discover how many tricks they have up their sleeves. Our job is to outsmart the genes.

That was the end of the story of Fred's drug-resistance work, because he had to finish his Ph.D., present his thesis, and move to a lab in Cambridge to study genes that make antibodies (immunoglobulin genes)—work in which Fred became a world authority. But gene amplification in cancer never left his mind. He reasoned that if cancer cells could amplify a gene to ward off a chemo drug, growth-control genes might be able to blossom in number to cause cancer in the first place.

No amplified genes had been identified that might cause cancer in human cells. Though Alt had become immersed in immunology in the Baltimore laboratory, he still wanted to find an example of a human oncogene. In 1978, he had an idea. He knew that the cells of one kind of pediatric cancer, neuroblastoma, had some extra bits of chromosomes that matched the additional bits in methotrexate-resistant cells. He ordered a bunch of neuroblastoma cell lines, and with Clifford Tabin, then a graduate student and now a professor of genetics at Harvard Medical School, he began studying whether the bits of chromosomes in them were related to some kind of cancer-causing gene.

At first, Alt and Tabin had poor luck. For some reason, they had received a bad batch of a chemical they needed as part of their experiment. Fred turned back to his main work in the Baltimore lab. He did not return to look for a possible amplification of genes in human cancer for another year or so, when he established his own lab at Columbia University.

Fred recalls, "In the meantime, probably a year earlier, a couple of guys from Mike Bishop's lab (where the term *oncogene* was coined) were randomly screening breast cancer lines and found that the growth-controlling gene myc was amplified in some tumors." Those researchers were the first to identify a human oncogene. Later, at Columbia, Fred and his collaborators discovered that a myc-like oncogene could become amplified and cause neuroblastoma in human cells. They named the gene N-myc.

"What we did not do, because we did not have access to clinicians, was immediately set up collaboration with a big consortium of clinicians working on neuroblastoma. It seemed fairly obvious that we should check the various stages of the disease and see if there was any correlation between the extent of amplification and disease stage. Mike Bishop and his group did that and found that the most aggressive neuroblastomas were the ones that had really high levels of the oncogene. That amplification totally correlated with prognosis. It was a great prognostic indicator."

Fred offers a story about the aftermath of his neuroblastoma discovery. "I was at a meeting in New York and got into a taxi. The taxicab driver asks, 'What do you do?' And I told him, 'I work in immunology and in cancer biology. We study how cancer cells get transformed.' And he said, 'Oh, you would be very interested in this.' He went on: 'Do you know that a bunch of guys just found out that this gene called N-myc is amplified in neuroblastoma and they can use it to judge how bad the disease is going to be?' This is a cab driver who tells me this. I just said, 'Really?' I never mentioned my role in it to that amazing New York cab driver."

Gene amplification is not the only cause of cancer. Other changes in genes can also lead to the disease. For example, excessive expression of a growth-promoting protein from a single growth-promoting gene (called a dominant oncogene) plays a role in many childhood leukemias, several lymphomas (tumors of lymph nodes), and multiple myeloma, a tumor of antibody-producing cells. The cancers develop because the growth-promoting gene is broken away from its normal resting place in the chromosome and fuses to a very strong promoter or enhancer of another gene. A similar but different mistake may occur in the leukemias and sarcomas, the cancers of supporting tissues like fibrous tissue, cartilage, and bone. A growth-promoting gene may fuse to another gene and change its DNA base sequence. This can create a hyperactive protein. (This is what happened to Mario's MLL gene.) Finally, a growth-promoting gene may develop a tiny point mutation that greatly raises the activity of that gene. I will describe more about some of these genetic accidents later in this book.

Fred Alt's work is a beautiful example of how curiosity-driven, basic research can lead to highly practical and applicable information about human disease. I wonder whether Fred would have stayed in immunology had the compound he needed to do his initial experiment on neuroblastoma worked properly. While he ended up leaving the field for several years, every oncology researcher is grateful for what he accomplished in the short time he devoted to this work. I always believed that he would one day return to the cancer problem and fortunately he has. His present work is on the cutting edge of cancer research.

The knowledge that Fred Alt generated about drug resistance in cancer had to influence Scott's thinking and the concerns of Steve Sallan and Lew Silverman about Mario. The MLL brand of childhood leukemia can develop resistance to therapy in many ways. If researchers could determine the specific Achilles' heel of the MLL tumor and define the metabolic pathway that the MLL malignant cell requires, then they might be able to design a smart drug to block it. Scott was determined to pursue that quest. Meanwhile, Mario had to be hit with a tidal wave of drugs for two months in the hospital, then go as an outpatient to the Jimmy Fund Clinic for a further two-year encounter with cocktails of broadly toxic drugs.

Scott's next job was to work out a plan with the nurses and the other staff to make that long encounter bearable for Mario and his family while he watched carefully for the emergence of drug resistance, the bane of cancer therapy.

CHAPTER SIX

# Three Critical Smart Drugs: Nursing Care, Psychology, and Social Work

The oncology ward at Children's Hospital, known as 7 West, was where Flavia and Walter had been educated about the risk of Mario developing chemotherapy resistance. They made every effort to abolish the thought, since they could not do anything to prevent it. They had accepted the highly toxic two-year treatment plan. Now they were directing all of their energy to everything they could do to help Mario—and survive the experience themselves.

Walter could sometimes escape because he worked during the day and slept at home at night. But Flavia lived with the pain, hour after hour, day after day, week after week. The differences in the couple's schedules, their sleeplessness and loss of intimacy, and their contrasting exposures to the high and low points of Mario's long hospitalization drove a subtle but palpable wedge between them.

The experienced nurses, psychologists, and social workers on 7 West saw that trouble coming and did what they could to prevent an unbridgeable chasm between Mario's parents. That response was also a smart drug to Mario and his family. Here was a kind of actual medicine that was not chemical but one that delivered vital emotional support. In recent years, emotional support has become increasingly recognized as critical in helping patients and families deal with the period of medical intervention involving cancer. In fact, several studies show that quality-of-life outcomes are far better for patients and families who receive appropriate emotional support during treatment. Furthermore, there is evidence that overall survival is improved as well.

Independently of such studies, the nurses worked to deliver Mario's care efficiently, safely, and above all, predictably, while doing what they could to support Flavia and Walter. Their attention to detail relieved Flavia, who understandably was watching everything, like a fish eagle guarding her nest. The psychological help that the care team provided to Mario and his parents undoubtedly helped all of them get through the harrowing two-month hospital stay.

Flavia and Walter were the second emotional smart drug that Mario received. For her part, Flavia slept or sat next to Mario, whether he was in his room or the playroom or the X-ray or radiotherapy clinic or the operating room for injections of chemotherapy into his spinal fluid. Walter never missed a meeting with physicians and nurses and came to the hospital daily, allowing Flavia to get some rest during the day.

Involved and thoughtful family members play critical roles in the emotional health of patients, especially children. Cancer in a child is a crisis that a family can only survive intact if it is tightly knit and focused on the effective treatment of the child. Nurses, psychologists, and social workers must be vigilant and detect stress faults that may crack the unity of parents, who are the key supporters of the child. When the fault lines are found, the care team must try to repair them by warm and sympathetic counseling that allows the parents to vent and release tension.

Other forms of tension release can be equally effective. Some years ago, a visiting German psychologist, an expert guitar player, asked me to allow him to play songs for the children and their parents during the evening. He had a beautiful voice and his guitar technique was quite magical. There was an obvious relaxing effect on the patients, the parents, and the staff. The tension on the ward disappeared when he was present. I hated to see him return to Germany.

Some patients simply have no family support, and they suffer even if the nurses and social workers do their very best to help them. Flavia knew all about such unfortunate children. Three years after Mario was admitted, she volunteered for a year at Children's Hospital and remarked, "I actually have seen kids who just sit there, and they don't have anybody. . . . Medicine has a big impact, but a family member's love is just as important. I have seen kids just be so lonely."

Other new medical devices have eased cancer treatment. One device, called a portacath, particularly helped Mario through chemotherapy. A portacath is a plastic container that is embedded under the skin of a patient's chest and attaches to a thin tube that connects to a large central vein. It permits the nurses to inject drugs without having to set up an IV directly into a vein every time chemotherapy is administered. In Mario's case, his nurses would numb the skin over the portacath with an anesthetic cream, then painlessly insert a needle bearing the drug into the container, from where it could go into the blood system. Only one or two years earlier, portacaths were thought to be too bulky for children of Mario's size. Mario went through most of that month with flying colors.

Mario vomited perhaps only twice from the chemo treatments that first month in the hospital. The multiple spinal taps presented more of a challenge. During the first one, three nurses, a doctor, and Flavia were needed to keep the child still. From that point on, the taps were always done in the operating room, with anesthesia. Mario then would always wake up after a tap and immediately say, "Mommy, I want ice." And within a half hour, he would start walking again. Mario's ability to bounce back seemed fine, which gave Flavia hope.

But then came radiation in the second month. "That was horrible," she recalled. Mario looks terrible in photos taken during that time. Still, his spirits were good enough that he was always smiling in those snapshots.

"You could really see him change—the transformation in his face and the loss of his hair," Walter added. Fortunately, however, Mario did not get any infections.

Next came Mario's transition from Children's Hospital to the Jimmy Fund Clinic at Dana-Farber. "I had looked forward to the end of the therapy in the hospital because I was so afraid that Mario would get an infection, and I knew the risk was highest in the first two months. But when the time came, it was tough to make that transition," Flavia said. "The hospital staff had become our family." She marveled about the support she received there. "I probably felt safer in the hospital than at home."

Nursing care for Mario and his mother also worked out well at the clinic. "I would not have made it without Annie, Mario's nurse there." As Flavia related this, she began to cry softly. "Annie Beauchemin was my rock. She would know what was going on with me right away just by looking at me. I knew she cared about me and how I felt."

Flavia's tribute to Mario's nurses at the hospital and the outpatient clinic is not unusual. Today, oncology nurses are trained to focus both on emotionally supporting the patient (and in pediatrics, the parents) and carrying out high-risk procedures such as administering chemotherapy, the orders for which must be checked multiple times. Good oncology nurses become near-magical figures to family members. They are very special people who devote themselves to the care of patients and families in dire distress. The emotional burdens that they carry would be too much for the average person. These nurses are not average. They have my undying respect and admiration.

Flavia and Walter also met repeatedly with Joanna Breyer, a highly experienced psychologist at the clinic who also helped to manage their needs in the hospital. "We really needed her," Flavia said. "The tension was so terrible—it was affecting our marriage. We were beginning to blame each other, and we each handled our sadness so differently. . . . Marriages are fragile to begin with, and young couples like us can be shattered by something like this." She pointed out that each family member copes with the threatened loss of a child in a unique way. Frictions always occur. It's very natural. "Joanna really helped us."

When we first spoke together, neither Flavia nor Walter were far from the pain they had endured after a very sick Mario had entered the hospital. Walter had come to the point at which he recognized that what he called the "nightmare" of childhood leukemia can come again anytime, frightening though that is. "We have to live with that uncertainty."

Flavia wiped her eyes with a tissue that was crushed in her hand. "I'm paying the consequences now. Right after Mario was out of treatment, I started to have all sorts of physical pain and aches," she said. "I need to let go of that constant fear of something happening to him."

Though she knew that the nurses were trained to detect evidence of relapse or other complications such as serious infections and that neither had occurred, she remained apprehensive that they would detect disaster on the next visit. Flavia had full confidence in Scott Armstrong, and she respected him for his skill in searching for adverse emotional consequences in parents who were struggling to maintain their hopes in the face of a dire medical threat to their child. She wanted to see him on her return visits to the clinic with Mario but dreaded what he might find. Annie Beauchemin somehow guided her through the emotional thicket.

Beauchemin came to Children's Hospital to work on the inpatient oncology unit in 1984, as soon as she completed four years of required experience in adult nursing in a large community hospital. She spent another four years at Children's before joining the Jimmy Fund Clinic at Dana-Farber, where she has worked ever since. She has seen many changes for the better, including the use of portacaths in young children, anesthetic creams before the insertion of an IV needle, and ondansetron (Zofran), a powerful antinausea medicine.

I have awe for Annie. She is remarkably open and honest. "Mario was a toddler and very typical of toddlers," Beauchemin told me. "They're afraid of doctors and nurses." The first times she needed to take a sample of Mario's blood through his portacath, she had to negotiate the boy's anxiety with a combination of patience, cajoling, and giving a bottom line. The technique worked. After several times, "Mario would run up to me. Then he'd climb on the table, sit there, and thrust his chest out, like, 'Okay, go ahead.'"

Annie also gave Mario his chemotherapy, which required giving him fairly painful injections into his fanny for twenty weeks in a row. That experience developed somewhat along the lines of Pavlov's work with dogs. Mario became accustomed to the routine because Annie never lied to him. If she said, "No shot," he knew she meant it. He also knew that if Beauchemin said, "Shot time," he had to accept what was coming.

Annie became very fond of Flavia. "She was terrified," the nurse recalled. They began to share much more than the mother's worries about the disease. They discussed basic parenting matters, such as how Mario could climb safely as he reached that developmental stage. In part, Beauchemin said, she thought the relationship grew as it did because Flavia felt somewhat isolated in her position, as an immigrant mother with an ill child.

"The one thing that's most important to impart [to parents] is that their child is special. I feel we need to relate to the families personally," Annie said. "I tell them what I did this weekend. It just makes them feel more comfortable, and it takes the pressure off of them." She has developed a method for handling parents' worries about their children. "For instance, when Mario's mother would look right into my heart and say,

'Is he doing okay?,' then I would try to put things in perspective by say-ing, 'At some point, I hope to be at his college graduation.' A few times, I had to say, 'What I have in front of me tells me that everything is fine today. I can't tell you more than that. We'll take one day at a time.' I was always honest with her."

At the time of my interview with Annie Beauchemin, Mario had completed his therapy and was still in complete remission three years after his original diagnosis. Both Annie and I knew that Mario still had a substantial chance of relapsing. The nurse was handling that informa-tion with Flavia and Walter as she did with all the parents who recognize that relapse is possible. "I treat everybody as though they are going to make it. Why come in with doom and gloom? That's not going to help anyone. And if sometime later the cancer should return, this perspective will have kept the parents from feeling that they spent every minute of every day waiting for the other shoe to drop. Cancer does not have to be the first thing that parents think of every morning when they get up."

And so she and Scott Armstrong have advised that Flavia and Wal-ter let Mario have a normal life. "He's a fine kid," said Annie. "Just let him grow up."

I've personally been spared the threat of a life-endangering illness in any of my children or grandchildren. But I have been close to many par-ents of seriously threatened children, and I know their agony. I do not believe that I could face that tension without the support of nurses like Annie and psychologists like Joanna. Yes—I would need the best of physicians in order to be confident that all was being done to save my beloved child. But even that confidence would not take me through the awful moments of doubt and terror. Those great nurses, psychologists, and social workers understand. They recognize the signs and symptoms of misery and they deal with them. They are smart drugs because they are the key to successful cancer therapy for children, and no one knows that better than Flavia and Walter.

Cancer treatment, particularly the treatment of children, is a multi-disciplinary team effort. And as is true of every team, each player is a vital member. Pediatric oncologists have known that fact for many years. Mario and his family came through their private purgatory because a fine team came to their aid.

# CHAPTER SEVEN

# Mario's Future

F lavia and Walter needed all the emotional support Mario's nurses, psychologists, and social workers could give them during their nearly two-year ordeal in the Jimmy Fund Clinic. But they made it through that time. Their marriage survived the enormous stress, and they never removed Mario from the educational track that they had always planned for him. When he turned three, he went to preschool every weekday except Mondays, his exhausting day at the clinic.

Walter spoke proudly as he recalled Mario's recovery and his early days in preschool.

"We put him into school. We started having him play soccer and all kinds of other things." While Mario sometimes lacked physical strength, he maintained his sense of confidence. Walter added, "This kid has resilience and a will about him that has amazed us."

Flavia agreed. "That's what Scott and Annie always told us. Just let him have a normal life. He's a fine kid."

They both became reflective as they recalled those terrible years. They remembered how they would badger Scott and the nurses after they came across something about new treatments for leukemia in the news media. Walter is multilingual and would scour the Internet in several languages. Every challenging nugget was presented to Scott for his opinion. Once Scott sighed that they were making him work for his money.

The two distraught young parents came to rely on Scott as a font of medical wisdom far beyond his years and experience. As is true of so many parents in their situation, they bound themselves to Scott, establishing a friendship with him. In some unconscious way, I believe, they wanted to link Scott to them so that he could never let Mario die. They had known children who had died on 7 West. Scott could never let that happen to Mario.

Flavia had retained her religious faith as well as her confidence in Scott. She knew that the real chances of Mario's survival were at best fifty-fifty, but she left it to God to decide—"whatever God thinks is right for my child."

Walter would rail at her religious beliefs. He had "used up" all his faith in the terrible process. He was angry at God. "If this is God, I don't want him." God was robbing him of his son's security. Walter found much more support in talking to parents who were in a similar plight. He could unburden to them because they knew what he was going through. He could even talk to them about his personal crises: he had lost his job and all of his health benefits just after Mario had been admitted. Fortunately he was able to apply successfully for Medicaid and achieved seamless coverage, but the humiliation added to the terrible strain of those endless days. Mario's illness, the savage impact of the treatment, the losses of jobs and health insurance, and the threat that they could not make payments on their apartment all contributed to a deep sense of insecurity and profound fear of the future. Flavia and Walter desperately needed to regain confidence, but they feared they would not until Mario could cross the five-year mark and still be free of disease.

The tension and the uncertainty got the best of Flavia for months after the two-year treatment period had ended and she no longer regularly saw Scott, Annie, and Joanna. She had to undergo expensive psychotherapy because she became preoccupied by morbid thoughts. "I was very depressed. I thought of death constantly—my own death from cancer and death in general. I kept asking when my death might come. I felt so very sick. I knew there was something terribly wrong with me. I begged for death to take me."

And Mario was uneasy, too. They could see that in his games. He would play endlessly with stuffed animals and set up intravenous lines with which to treat them. He said that they would die if he didn't give them the needles.

At the three-year mark, they began to breathe a little. Flavia had rid herself of her morbid thoughts and planned to return to work part-time and then full-time in her commercial art career. Walter got a temporary job. Flavia told me, "We have Mario. All three of us have to recover our lives."

I saw Flavia several months later. Mario had just turned six and had been free of leukemia for four years. I noted that she looked far less care-worn and asked her if she felt as well as she looked.

She responded enthusiastically. "Oh, yes—I am beginning to breathe again. Walter just needs to get a good permanent job and I'll be able to believe that we are going to be on our way back. I'm looking hard for work myself." In 2004, Mario passed the five-year mark in excellent health, and both Flavia and Walter were fully employed. In 2005, at the six-year mark, Flavia brought Mario to see me. He was a good-looking seven-year-old. No one would ever guess that he had been gravely ill. His chances of relapse are now quite low. Flavia and Walter believe that he will grow up to become a wonderful young man. He is still in remission in late 2006.

As Flavia and Walter were trying to regain their lives and Mario was progressing in school, Scott Armstrong had started his laboratory research program in 2002 focusing on MLL. He still maintained Mondays as his weekly commitment to the follow-up care of his patients and served for two months a year as the supervising physician on the oncology inpatient and consultation services. He devoted the rest of his time to laboratory research efforts. This is the classical career of the physician scientist. But as a scientist, Scott wanted his research to be about patients. That's why he chose MLL.

To pursue the cure for MLL, Scott wisely chose to work in the laboratory of the late Stanley Korsmeyer at Dana-Farber. Korsmeyer, a physician and leading basic scientist, had been working on and off on the MLL translocation in infant leukemia for a decade. He had determined that in MLL leukemia a normal gene that he called the MLL gene is altered by a chromosomal rearrangement or translocation that changes the structure of the gene into one that makes a hyperactive MLL protein. That hyperactive MLL protein in turn holds other genes that are in the state of making protein in the "on" position. Some of those genes, Korsmeyer reasoned, must help to drive the leukemia. But Korsmeyer did not know why infant leukemia was so pernicious and difficult to treat, and he was eager to know how the hyperactive MLL protein rendered lymphocytes so persistently malignant.

Scott's interest in MLL matched Korsmeyer's perfectly, and Scott was welcomed into the Korsmeyer lab with enthusiasm. There he decided to pose the questions that Korsmeyer had been asking for a decade: What does hyperactive MLL protein do to make a lymphocyte malignant? Though hyperactive MLL protein surely affects scores of genes and holds them in the "on" or protein-producing state, which ones are the important offenders?

Scott decided to collaborate with Todd Golub, one of his colleagues in pediatric oncology. Todd, then an assistant professor of pediatrics at Dana-Farber and Harvard Medical School and a few years older than Scott, had rapidly become one of the world leaders in the assessment of the genes that are turned on to make protein or are shut down in leukemic and other cancer cells. Like Korsmeyer, Todd had begun his oncology research career by examining the translocations that cause cancers of the blood and lymphatic system. His initial interest was childhood leukemia. He had been the discoverer of the translocation that causes a fusion of two genes, tel and aml1, which inactivates the tel gene. In sharp contrast to MLL, the tel/aml1 gene fusion is associated with an excellent prognosis. In fact, in 1999, when Mario was first admitted, Golub, his mentor, Gary Gilliland of the Brigham and Women's Hospital, and Steven Sallan had found that 100 percent of children with a tel/aml1 fusion resulting from a translocation between chromosomes 12 and 21 had been cured by Sallan's treatment protocol. But Golub had wanted to delve further into the roots of the genetic problems in childhood leukemia and measure the output of all of the twenty thousand to twenty-five thousand human genes that might be overexpressed, normally expressed, or deficiently expressed in the various forms of childhood leukemia. MLL leukemia would be a good place to start.

Examination of the expression of twenty-five thousand genes sounds like an enormous task. With standard methods, the task would require dozens of scientists working for years. But Golub and his collaborator, Eric Lander, a professor of biology at MIT and now the director of the Broad Institute at MIT and Harvard, had decided to take a huge shortcut called gene expression profiling by microarray analysis, which had been proposed by scientists at the Geron Corporation in California and was in the process of commercial development. It would require some excellent computer-assisted data management and the application of robotic technology, but those were relatively simple matters for Lander, who had morphed from a career in econometrics into biology and had been a leading member of the national effort to decode the human genome. What Lander did not have were examples of human diseases in which the new technology could be applied; nor did he have a colleague who understood both the diseases and the technology. He found that happy amalgam in Golub. By 1999, the year before Scott Armstrong started in Korsmeyer's laboratory, Golub and Lander were making major progress in the dissection of gene expression in the leukemias. The stage was set for a major collaborative study of MLL.

Events moved very quickly. Armstrong had many samples of MLL cells that had been derived from the therapeutic collaboration established by Sallan and Silverman with their colleagues in the Netherlands and in Toronto. ALL (acute lymphoblastic leukemia) and AML (acute myeloblastic leukemia) cells were readily available in the freezers of Dana-Farber. Golub measured the thousands of messenger RNAs produced by their genes. To the excitement of all of the collaborators, the three leukemias were readily distinguished on the basis of their gene expression. Looking through the microscope and guessing at differences by appearance had been totally supplanted. It was now very clear that MLL and AML are more difficult to treat than standard ALL because the former express the same twenty-five thousand human genes in different proportions. And MLL is readily distinguished from AML on the same basis. The three diseases look roughly the same, but they express their genes in unique patterns. Scott, Golub, and others later showed that the hyperactive MLL gene turns normal bone marrow cells into cells that can continuously divide; in effect, they become cancer stem cells. That is why MLL is so hard to treat.

But there was even more to come. Armstrong and Golub decided to rank the genes that seemed to be favored for high expression by MLL cells. One gene popped up immediately from their survey. It was flt3, a gene that produces a protein called receptor tyrosine kinase. Flt3 would, if overexpressed, make high amounts of protein and be expected to drive cells to grow continuously. In some other MLL samples, flt3 was expressed at a normal rate, but the enzyme was mutated to be much more highly active. Clearly the flt3 gene and its protein were potential villains in MLL.

Those discoveries immediately opened up other major collaborations, this time with James Griffin, the chief of medical oncology and a

colleague right down the hall who had been studying the growth of leukemia cells for years, and with another young colleague, Andrew Kung,
a pediatric oncologist who had developed a new model system for measuring the growth of human leukemia cells in rodents.

Griffin had already found that flt3 could be responsible for the
excessive growth of AML cells in adults. He was collaborating with scientists at Merck who had found a smart drug they called PKC412 that
binds to flt3 protein and abolishes its activity. In 2003, Kung treated mice
transplanted with MLL cells and found that the leukemia was totally
arrested by PKC412. A magic bullet of the kind envisioned fifty-five
years earlier by Sidney Farber had been found for children with leukemia. Scott Armstrong, who had begun his career in pediatric oncology
with a clinical interest in MLL, had performed a translation of basic science into clinical medicine that is sought after by many aspiring young
physician scientists but rarely achieved. His work received high acclaim,
was broadly recognized, and was awarded with significant prizes as well
as research grants. He soon established his own independent laboratory
and was promoted to become an assistant professor of pediatrics at Harvard Medical School.

Scott is clearly on the way to a successful career. But he knows that he
owes it all to his patients like Mario and to the many colleagues who had
collaborated with him. They, in turn, know that Scott is a physician scientist highly worthy of collaboration. He has the drive, the determination,
and the sharing attitude that makes collaboration a joy instead of a trial.

Mario is doing brilliantly. He bears no sign of leukemia, and he has
crossed the six-year mark in complete remission. He is very likely to be
one of the fortunate 50 percent who does well on the new aggressive
AraC/high-dose methotrexate protocol. But if he relapses, Scott has the
flt3 inhibitor, a smart drug, as another arrow in his therapeutic options.
As we will learn in Ken's story, receptor tyrosine kinase inhibition by
smart drugs is currently the hot topic in cancer therapy. It is a remarkable innovation and one that would make Sidney Farber say, "I told you
so," but it is not perfect. Cancer cells become resistant to the new drugs.
We have to find a way around that serious problem.

Nonetheless, Mario's story clearly demonstrates that the childhood
leukemias, even the most severe cases, can be conquered. We have moved
from an era of hopelessness in the 1950s to an era of huge accomplish-
ment in the first part of the twenty-first century. Medical progress may be

slower than we want, but it is inexorable, and a new class of smart drugs is on the horizon. That progress requires deep commitment by patients, physicians, basic scientists, nurses, pharmacists, other vital supporting staff, and the pharmaceutical industry. It also requires commitment by the public represented by the trustees of research-oriented institutions and foundations and by dedicated government agencies. By making a commitment to Mario and to patients like him, we make the progress recounted in his story—as I have seen unfold from the unmitigated gloom of my own medical student days to the high promise of the present.

# Joan's Story

# CHAPTER EIGHT

# A Pleasant Summer Day

O ne morning in the summer of 2000, I elbowed my way into line at our small village newsstand. In my haste to get a newspaper, I almost failed to notice Joan. She's not a pusher or a shover. The daily struggle for New York newspapers brings out the worst in well-heeled vacationers. If those transplanted city folk cannot get a copy of the *Times* and the *Wall Street Journal*, their vastly overpriced coffees and croissants will be nearly tasteless. Joan, in contrast, likes to take life in the village as it comes. She's more interested in the ambience than in a particular possession. She comes to the store after her morning walk with "the girls," her friends of many years, to get coffee and perhaps the *Times* if it's available. If it's not, so much the better. "There is plenty of opportunity to hear bad news these days," she says.

On this occasion, Joan wanted to talk to me. She asked if I would have a few moments to discuss a personal issue that had just emerged. In her quiet, undemanding way, she wondered whether I would be able to chat with her sometime during the day. The fact is that I would be delighted to chat with Joan any day at any time. She and her husband, Bob, are summer friends. We've known each other for decades. Bob and I used to play a fierce game of singles. He had both skill and determination. I lacked the former and emphasized the latter. We would emerge from the court soaked and breathless, vowing to do better next time. Then Bob developed a tennis back and we transferred our battles to the golf course, where they still go on.

Joan loves to walk in the early morning, and she enjoys our foursome on the golf course because it provides a beautiful stroll on rolling hills with many glimpses of the sea and its magnificent signature lighthouse that stands precariously on an eroding cliff. Hitting the ball is another matter. None of us do that very well. Bob and I take our many failures on the course somewhat to heart. Joan seems to be content to look forward to a pleasant walk during which she hopes to find her ball. If she gets off a particularly terrible shot, she will say, "That didn't happen," and hit another one. We keep score by approximation. At least when I play with her, her handicap and all the excruciatingly dull details of golf seem far from her mind.

Joan and I walked the few blocks from the store to my house on the edge of the village chatting about her efforts to focus the minds and energies of the summer residents on the environmental pressures that threaten our idyllic vacation existence. Joan is a community worker. She just can't avoid that responsibility, even on vacation. She was born and raised in eastern Ohio in a middle-class home in which education and responsibility for all of the members of one's family and larger community were the highest ideals. Joan taught high school near her hometown for several years but always looked for ways to participate in efforts to make improvements in local social services. She wants her life to make a difference for individuals and broader communities.

Joan met Bob at a church social and knew immediately that he would be the man for her. An avid basketball player, he had soon seen that there are saner ways to make a living. He had moved up the corporate ladder in a large company in Georgia, but he wanted to go into business for himself. He decided to set up shop in a town in central Massachusetts. There the two of them settled down in a comfortable suburb and started a family and business. They flourished.

Joan continued to teach school and focus on community improvements in the town. Bob's business provides fire prevention services for corporations, hospitals, and stores throughout western New England and upper New York State. It is a big and demanding territory that has to be carefully supervised. Though there are plenty of employees, Bob is in charge of the analysis of fire risk to businesses in which his equipment is in place. He has to be ready to travel if something somewhere doesn't work. If there is a fire in a building in which his equipment is utilized, Bob's life can become hectic.

By dint of hard work and attention to detail, the business has succeeded. Joan and Bob and their two children, Ellen and Jeff, have enjoyed summer vacations near my home, which is how I met them.

Joan developed a curriculum to train students in kindergarten through high school to appreciate community service, with internships in various voluntary and town government agencies. Her work drew national attention and recently led to a prestigious appointment to a federal government commission that supports the national effort in community service.

Joan doesn't look her age. That morning, she appeared much younger than sixty-two, dressed in a short-sleeved shirt, walking shorts, and athletic shoes. After we sat on my porch well away from the crowd, she brushed her light hair back with her hand and started to talk about what had happened in her life in late July.

Joan and Bob were particularly happy that month. They had finally decided to build a house near the summer village that we enjoy so much. With difficulty, they had found the right piece of land; construction was progressing so well that they thought they would be able to be in the new house before the following summer. The house would be comfortable, possibly for retirement. Joan could see that possibility on the not-too-distant horizon. Jeff had joined the company. In time, he might learn the business well enough to take it over. Ellen had just gotten married and was living near the village with her husband.

During one of the house-planning sessions, Joan leaned on a table to make rough drawings and noticed that the nipple of her left breast was discharging fluid. She had noted the same discharge a month earlier and had visited a dermatologist, who biopsied the nipple and concluded that she had eczema. He gave her a cream for it.

She went upstairs to examine her breast. It was lumpy as usual, but there were no new lumps that Joan could detect. She considered herself fairly skillful at breast self-examination. Her cystic breasts had demanded close attention and frequent mammograms ever since her fiftieth birthday.

There was a striking cancer background in Joan's family. Her mother had died of ovarian cancer, and two of her mother's sisters and one brother had died of other cancers. Both daughters of her father's brother have had breast cancer. But Joan's strong family history of breast and ovarian cancer, while faintly consistent with the presence of a cancer susceptibility gene, was more likely due to chance. As far as recent research has been able to show, inherited cancer is very rare.

Joan had never smoked, was not obese, did not abuse alcohol, and gave birth to her children in her late twenties. Hence there were no obvious risks for breast cancer in her background except for one: she had taken hormone replacement pills ever since the onset of her menopause and continued them for twelve years. Two months prior to her discussion with me, Joan had discontinued hormone replacement because she had learned that the treatment increases the risk of breast cancer.

Joan felt her breasts carefully. She positioned them just as she had been taught by her gynecologist and gently probed with her fingers trying to find a new lump. She knew her lumps by heart, and there was nothing new that she could detect this time. She could find nothing that had not been palpable for months or even years. But she admitted to herself that she might miss a new lump in her complex breast structure. With a resigned sigh, she picked up the phone and called her gynecologist for an appointment. She did not tell Bob about the discharge or about her decision to schedule the appointment.

# CHAPTER NINE

# Bad News

The gynecologist wasn't sure. She squeezed Joan's breast. A small drop of fluid appeared on the nipple. She probed each breast with a practiced hand and after several minutes concluded that they felt about the same. There seemed to be a little larger area of lumpiness at the base of the left breast, but the lumps had been there for years and the gynecologist was unimpressed with her own examination. She told Joan that she was sure there were no changes, but she suggested further tests.

Physical examination of the breast to detect cancers is a ritualistic part of a woman's medical evaluation. In fact, women in the United States who have normal blood pressure and are younger than sixty are far more at risk of the sum of breast, cervix, and thyroid cancer than any other problem including coronary disease. A careful examination to detect an early breast, thyroid, or cervical cancer is absolutely mandatory. Yet most internists are not very well trained to perform such exams. That's why women should see a gynecologist once a year. But there are serious questions about the role of the physical examination in early detection of these cancers, particularly in women who have lumpy breasts. Even gynecologists who regularly examine breasts admit that lumps due to fibrocystic changes, which often cause nodules in otherwise perfectly healthy breast tissue, are difficult to categorize. And only overconfident gynecologists would make the claim that they can detect the difference between a cystic lump and a cancerous lump with any degree of reliability.

Women between the ages of twenty and forty may also have hard-to-examine breasts due to a high density of fibrous tissue and the onset of fibrocystic changes. The fibrotic strands hold the breast in its position at right angles to the chest. As the fibrous tissue disappears with age, the breast begins to gain fat and sag. It's a relief for the examiner because the breast becomes much smoother and softer, and small areas of hardness that could be cancers are more detectable in the hands of those who know how to find them. The fibrocystic changes that occur in at least 50 percent of women are the physiological results of hormone alterations, not illness.

A qualified examiner who keeps careful records, has a patient with soft nodule-free breasts, and examines those breasts carefully every year can and does pick up early cancer. The problem is that suspicious nodules when biopsied often turn out to be benign. That subjects some patients to unnecessary procedures.

Nonetheless, early detection saves lives and improves quality of life because breast cancer that is diagnosed early is highly curable with minimally invasive therapy and often with no chemotherapy. At least 80 percent of women with small invasive breast cancers that are restricted to the breast can be cured with simple lumpectomy to which breast irradiation, intended to kill cancer cells undetected in the surgical margins, is usually added to prevent local recurrence.

Given the uncertainty of the results of the physical examination in women with the kinds of fibrocystic changes that Joan had in her breasts, the gynecologist recommended a mammogram, a decision that launched Joan into a whirlwind. Joan is a careful person. Her house is immaculate. She comes from a conservative family that taught her to do important things cautiously and correctly. She is thoughtful about her health. Most physicians would consider her the perfect patient—one who gives relevant information, asks intelligent questions, follows instructions, and keeps her physician informed. She was startled by the uncertainty of the events that followed.

The radiologist who performed Joan's mammogram added an ultrasound examination of both breasts in order to gain further understanding of the nodules at the base of Joan's left breast. Ultrasonography can be useful in the diagnosis of nodules because it differentiates fluid-filled cysts from solid nodules, the latter more likely to be cancers than manifestations of fibrocystic changes. Joan complied, and without telling Bob anything about her visit to her gynecologist or the imaging studies, she had both procedures in the radiology department of the hospital.

Of all of the improvements in diagnostic medicine that I have observed in the past fifty years, none are more remarkable and valuable than those contributed by the imaging sciences. Fifty years ago, we could do routine X-rays of the chest and abdomen, and we could do certain studies with contrast media that absorbed X-rays and allowed indirect visualization of the kidneys and the intestines. Today, the advent of computer-assisted tomography (CAT or CT scan), magnetic resonance imaging (MRI), functional MRI, and positron emission tomography (PET scan) has revolutionized diagnosis. Not only can we see anatomical variations that were invisible before, but we can also observe the actual metabolism or function of tissues or even tumors before and after treatment. And if we want to obtain a sample of tissue with a biopsy needle, we can be guided directly to our target with ultrasound and obtain the sample with minimal hazard to the patient. Even routine examination of blood cells smeared on a glass slide, formerly the province of a trained microscopist, is performed by new imaging analyzers that can recognize patterns and discriminate the classes of cells. Technicians are trained to operate the machines as well as look at the cells.

The shadows cast on an X-ray film and the bulky envelopes of films that were regularly lost in radiology departments are being replaced by digitally stored records that can be called up by keyboards, placed on viewing screens, and transferred around the world on the Internet in seconds. Clinical imaging science is a very high-tech meeting place of clinicians, information scientists, and engineers who have revolutionized diagnostic medicine. But it's fair to say that one area lagging behind these dazzling advances in imaging technology is screening mammography.

For that procedure, Joan stood while her breasts were squeezed flat onto an X-ray film—from front to back and side to side. Then X-rays were delivered through her flattened breasts and collected on the film. Dense nodules would absorb more X-rays than normal tissue, and an experienced reader of the film could presumably determine breast cancer.

Joan's ultrasound analysis was straightforward. The cysts at the base of her left breast had enlarged somewhat. As simple cysts, they were not a matter of concern. Joan remained in the waiting room to learn the results of the mammogram.

Screening mammography has become the cornerstone of breast cancer prevention. Millions of women have screening mammograms every year if they are in health plans that provide them. Poor women or women in inadequate health insurance plans may not have them nearly as often as they should despite well-intentioned government programs. Some hospitals and cancer centers try to correct that inequity by sending mobile mammogram units into poor neighborhoods to screen as many women as possible in vans parked in neighborhoods or outside workplaces. Volunteers who climb the stairs of subsidized housing units in an effort to induce women at risk to have mammograms act as the persuaders. Clearly there is a strong belief that regular mammography saves lives. It can detect early breast cancer that would be missed by self-examination or physical examination by a physician.

Not surprisingly, the conclusion that mammography is lifesaving has been disputed. In fact, the cost-benefit value of screening tests to prevent illness of any kind is always disputed, as it should be. Whenever we adopt a screening test, we have to know its cost and its reliability. Only then can we calculate its value and decide whether to add it to our enormous health care budget.

The dispute over mammography has centered on its reliability. Does it reveal cancers that were not diagnosed by physical examination or does it miss most tumors, instead turning up a lot of false positives that lead to more invasive or expensive tests and few firm diagnoses? Does it really save lives? There is good reason to be suspicious. Mammograms are hard to read, particularly in young women whose breasts have fibrous tissue and in middle-aged women whose breasts are more fatty but may have fibrocystic changes. Mammograms cannot reliably distinguish cysts from nodules, but they can detect flecks of calcium in the breast that may be associated with cancer. They are more reliable than physical examinations, but the question is how much.

A respected pair of Danish investigators conducted a recent study of a large number of mammogram tests on women over the age of forty, utilizing a statistical method called meta-analysis. They threw out studies that they considered faulted by poor mammography technique and concluded that mammograms are of doubtful value. They merely cause expensive, invasive, and often unnecessary procedures because there are so many false positives. In fact, it is well established that somewhere between 30 and 50 percent of women who have had ten mammograms have a false positive examination that leads to an unnecessary biopsy. The Danish analysis and the high false positive rate have soured a number of experts in preventive medicine on mammography. But other experts reviewing the same studies have come to opposite conclusions.

The National Cancer Institute's special advisory groups on mammography have carefully considered the studies and have generally supported mammography screening for women over forty. The American Cancer Society has reiterated its stand that mammography is the only reasonable screening test that we have for breast cancer and we must use it. But the proponents of mammography screening (and I am one) have to recognize and should explain to their patients that annual mammograms reduce the risk of mortality from breast cancer by only about 20 percent if you look at the entire published literature objectively. And since the risk of mortality from treated breast cancer is not very high, the absolute reduction attributed to mammography is quite low, perhaps no better than 4 percent.

The dispute over mammography has been very unsettling not only for women like Joan but also for physicians who pride themselves on offering evidence-based medicine to their patients. A reasonable working conclusion for the individual physician and her patient is that mammography can be a valuable screening test in the hands of a very good mammographer reviewing the serial mammograms of a woman (particularly a woman over fifty) who has her annual mammograms in the same office year after year. The disputed studies may be seriously contaminated by the fact that such continuity is rarely achieved. So an individual physician like Joan's gynecologist depends on the quality of service provided by her colleagues in radiology and by the continuity offered by serial mammograms. But Joan's case illustrates the subtlety of the problem.

After a thirty-minute wait, the radiology technician who performed the mammogram came out to the waiting room to tell Joan there were some changes in her left breast, which the radiologist wanted to aspirate with a needle to see if fluid could be obtained. The aspiration attempt was unsuccessful; no fluid could be aspirated from the presumed cyst, and Joan was asked to return for a second visit when the most experienced mammographer would be present to review the films. She did return a few days later for another ultrasound and mammogram and sat down again to wait. The news was decidedly different. The experienced mammogram radiologist had carefully examined several of Joan's annual mammograms and compared them with the new ones. Kindly and gently, he told her that there was indeed a new and suspicious area of density in the left breast that was not there before. He recommended a fine-needle biopsy of that new area and arranged an appointment with a surgeon to do the procedure and to advise Joan about other biopsy alternatives.

Joan does not get disturbed easily. But while this second opinion in the same office actually represented excellent care, it made her apprehensive and very conscious of the randomness of interpretation. That radiology office is known to be first class and the physicians who staff it of the highest quality. But to Joan there seemed to be too much uncertainty.

Of course, if a screening test is to be usefully applied on a broad scale, it has to be reasonably easy to interpret. Otherwise, it can be applied effectively only to those who have access to the best and most carefully applied technology with radiologists who have the background and training that enables them to interpret the films correctly. Joan's experience should only serve to heighten the awareness of individual physicians and patients regarding the justifiable concern about the reliability of mammography, thus encouraging them to demand the very best technique when the time for annual screening or the need for a special study arises. Furthermore, patients have to understand that there will be false positives and accept that risk.

The desire for quality and convenience and the doubts about mammography have led to a surge in the development of private imaging offices by entrepreneurial radiologists in most U.S. cities and suburbs. A quick glance at the offerings on the Internet gives the whole picture.

Joan's unsettling experience of the mammogram gave her confidence a jolt, but she kept the appointment to have a biopsy of the suspicious area with the general surgeon recommended by the radiologist. The radiologist was quite confident that the surgeon could biopsy the correct area without ultrasound assistance. Without telling Bob anything about these developments, Joan had the procedure.

The surgeon was skillful. After he disinfected the skin of the breast, he inserted a very fine-caliber biopsy needle directly into the area in question and withdrew a tiny sliver of tissue only double the width of a human hair. There was no bleeding, but he placed a Band-Aid over the invisible hole and asked Joan to return in three days so that he could check the "wound" and go over the biopsy results, which he promised would be returned promptly by the efficient pathology department of the hospital.

Three days later, Joan returned to see the surgeon, who had the news that she had hoped she would not hear. The tiny wound was clean, but the biopsy revealed cancer cells. There was no doubt about the diagnosis. Joan would face the hard choices that confront so many women: choices about surgery of the breast and the breast-draining lymph nodes in the space under the arm called the axilla, hormone receptor blockade, radiation therapy, and chemotherapy. Joan liked the surgeon and appreciated his frankness. She told him that she would return after she had broken the news to her husband.

That evening, Joan sat in the living room waiting for Bob to come home. He was later than usual because he had traveled that day to upstate New York to establish space for a new branch office. As he entered the door, a heavy briefcase full of fire hazard specifications in his left hand and keys in his right, Joan called out to him.

"Bob, could we talk right away? I have something to tell you. I have breast cancer."

Bob stared straight ahead. He put down the heavy briefcase and looked dazedly up the stairwell. Without a word, he walked slowly up to the second floor. Joan was stunned. In what seemed to be an eternity but was only a few seconds, Bob almost ran down the stairs and into the living room, sat next to Joan, and hugged her closely.

"I hear you, Joan dear. I hear you now."

Bob's reaction to the totally unexpected news is a classic example of the human emotional defense system at work. When faced with imminent disaster, many of us simply shut down our senses. We neither see nor hear. We freeze. This occurs as well in the animal kingdom. A gazelle caught by a lion will stand still in its final seconds. It seems to shut off its entire brain rather than endure the horror. Bob's reaction was right out of a psychology textbook. He had the advantage of being preoccupied by serious business issues, but the shock of the news was the major force that temporarily dislodged him. He turned off his receptors and briefly departed the field. In seconds it all sank in, and he returned to the battle scene, never to leave it again.

CHAPTER TEN

# An Initial Plan

Joan quietly recounted her diagnosis to me and asked for my advice about the next steps in her care. I am a hematologist with a specialty in pediatric hematology, not an expert in the management of adults with breast cancer. But Joan knew that at that time I was the CEO of the Dana-Farber Cancer Institute and had just undertaken a substantial revision of many of its clinical and research programs. So she was confident that I would know highly trained and experienced physicians who focus all of their efforts on breast cancer.

The excellent general surgeon who had biopsied her breast was prepared to take the next steps to treat her. She liked and trusted that surgeon, and his office was a few moments from her house. Should she have her treatment at home in her own surroundings or come to Dana-Farber for a second opinion with the possibility of having her management assumed by the Dana-Farber Women's Cancers Program?

The question of best treatment options is one that has troubled me for decades. My first encounter with breast cancer and its potential ravages occurred during my early training in the late 1950s at the National Cancer Institute. I saw scores of young women with far advanced disease for whom there was no hope at all. The changes for the better in the past half century have been remarkable, particularly for postmenopausal women and even for younger women with estrogen receptor–positive breast cancer, which had been historically difficult to treat. The whole experience has made me consider how serious illness should be managed and who should manage it. How do we define "best" medical care? The question goes well beyond Joan's particular case and the specific issue of breast cancer. It opens up a consideration of the way we manage life-threatening disorders in the United States.

The answer depends so much on availability of alternatives. We have no organized system of regional medical care for major illness in the United States. Four decades ago, the Lyndon Johnson administration tried to establish such a system at least for heart disease, cancer, and stroke, but it fell by the wayside. The National Cancer Institute has partially funded sixty-one cancer centers around the country, thirty-nine of which are designated as comprehensive, meaning they offer state-of-the-art clinical and research programs in the common cancers that appear in all age groups. The comprehensive centers are assigned "responsibility" for certain regions. For example, the Dana-Farber Cancer Institute has putative responsibility for the care of cancer patients undergoing clinical trials in Massachusetts and Maine. But the responsibility is ephemeral because health care delivery is driven almost entirely by independent choice makers. There are the relatively few patients who have such broad health insurance coverage that they can go where they please for services. These are usually the executives of companies that offer top perks to their leaders and many government officers including all members of Congress. The rest of us have, in the recent past, gone where our employer-based managed care health plans allowed us to go. The decisions made by these health plans were occasionally based on quality but almost always on cost.

The arbitrary decisions of managed care health plans are relaxing somewhat today, but the decline in coverage by employers is still forcing those who are fortunate enough to have any insurance at all to seek care based on cost. That is certainly not all bad, but since no one, including our primary physician, is apt to tell us about the best option with complete objectivity, we usually do not know. Some managed care insurance companies and Medicare are actually publishing "objective" data about the quality of various health care providers, but the data are much too unreliable to be useful.

Oddly enough, the urban poor and uninsured, who get sick with higher frequency because they have limited or no access to preventive services, may get excellent care when they get serious diseases because they frequently end up in the emergency wards of our inner-city teaching hospitals, some (but not all) of which have cutting-edge clinical programs in the diseases that befall those patients. The rural poor (and there are many of them) are not as lucky. They have poor access to preventive *and* therapeutic programs. They are the most profound victims of our chaotic so-called system.

Those of us who have excellent primary physicians committed to our wellness should count our blessings. But our primary physicians are usually affiliated with local community hospitals and will be influenced to advise us to have our specialty care in those institutions because they have longstanding associations with the local specialists and want to keep the beds full in those hospitals. You may try to use the Internet as an adjunct to the advice of your primary physician, but the Internet is an unreliable source of information unless you are experienced enough to know exactly where to go and what page to open. It is really a large advertising medium for health care entrepreneurs. Major cancer centers may actually advertise in national media in order to attract patients away from their local community hospitals or from competing cancer centers, but patients are often worried about such advertisements. If cancer centers are so famous and so excellent, why do they need to advertise?

With respect to the common cancers like lung, breast, and bowel cancers, the problem is really very complex. There is no question that cutting-edge knowledge of care and clinical research in these cancers is far more likely to be found in designated cancer centers than in most community hospitals, even though many of the oncologists in community hospitals have received all or part of their training in cancer centers. But expertise does not always translate into better care. It is sometimes argued that care is better in designated cancer centers than in community hospitals because cancer center patients are more frequently enrolled in clinical trials. Actually, recent studies do not support the notion that enrollment in clinical trials necessarily improves outcome. Better outcome depends on whether the new approach investigated in a trial achieves a substantial improvement over standard therapy. Most of the time, it does not. Furthermore, some community hospitals avidly pursue clinical trials sponsored by pharmaceutical companies and their agents. These trials are of variable quality.

Some believe that designated cancer centers are apt to have better results because the quality of medical care is consistently proportional to volume. Experience counts in medical care. In fact, experience is probably the most important indicator of quality. This should be obvious.

After all, in a reasonably free system, the best will receive most of the referrals and will therefore enjoy the highest volume. But even that axiom does not always hold up to close scrutiny. Excellent outcomes in complex diseases *should* be proportional to volume, but the relationship is not linear and there are major exceptions.

There is another issue about cancer care that bubbles just below the surface. Managed care insurance companies and particularly Medicare tightly regulate the reimbursement of community oncologists and NCI-designated cancer centers. Oncologists, no matter where they practice, are not appropriately reimbursed for their time. They used to make money in their diagnostic laboratories, but laboratory tests are no longer reimbursed very well.

The sole source of profit for community oncologists or cancer centers turns out to be anticancer drug infusions. The community oncologists try to buy the drugs wholesale and charge above retail for their infusion. The profit pays for the oncologist's time. Medicare has recently lowered the boom on that financial practice by refusing to pay more than standard wholesale prices for drugs. Only large cancer centers can negotiate with drug companies to purchase drugs below standard wholesale prices. Smaller practices cannot do that very readily.

Since cancer is an age-dependent disease, most cancer patients are on Medicare. The result is a financial disaster for community oncologists, who may even overuse expensive radiology tests like MRIs that are well reimbursed in order to collect some money for a visit. In desperation, some community oncologists are trying to rid themselves of Medicare patients. The designated cancer centers survive not only because they can negotiate lower than standard wholesale drug prices from drug companies, but also because they can raise money from donors. This is another example of the tattered fabric of health care in the United States. There will soon be a massive outcry unless it is repaired.

Despite clinical and financial uncertainties, loyalty to the local institution remains a very strong force in American medical care. After the Second World War, we poured countless millions of Hill-Burton Act–generated and privately donated dollars into the construction of community hospitals. We also created hundreds if not thousands of specialty training programs to develop physicians capable of delivering evidence-based medicine. Most of those highly trained specialists could not find positions in the training centers and flooded the community hospitals.

Soon those hospitals, initially designed to deal with very common illnesses, were competing with the training centers for rare patients who require high-tech care because our medical reimbursement system is based
on payment for procedures rather than for actual time spent in the care
process.

A rash of purchases of community hospitals ensued and even physician practices by big training hospitals, many of which went into near
receivership as they parted with their precious cash in a tightening medical market. Then some very prominent training centers, advised by consultants swollen with hubris, concluded that they could not fight the
trend alone. They began to consolidate, adding the debts of one to the
negative cash flow of another, apparently with the bizarre idea that two
losses create a gain. The result has been serious erosion of the financial
security of some major cancer and cardiovascular treatment and research
centers. This bad judgment was balanced by an ever-tightening reimbursement system that began to drive the community hospitals under
water as well. The whole system has been awash in a musical chair game
of debt and fiscal uncertainty, with only a few megacontenders left
standing.

So Joan's question of where to have her treatment has to be answered
in the context of a system that is hideously expensive, poorly administered, and grossly uneven in quality. And even if all breast cancer patients
should be managed in a comprehensive cancer center, such a plan is
manifestly absurd because breast cancer, unlike childhood leukemia, is
too common to be managed in one place. Dana-Farber simply doesn't
have enough space or financial resources devoted to its Women's Cancers Program to manage more than a small fraction of the region's breast
cancer patients on site. Joan had to decide whether she wanted to consult
a very highly experienced breast cancer specialist in a cancer center and
make her therapeutic plans based on that visit or whether her more fundamental need was to be at home, not a hundred miles away from friends
and family. My own bias was fairly obvious. I thought she should seek a
second opinion at Dana-Farber and then make up her mind.

That evening, Joan met with three of her closest summer friends, all
of whom had had to deal with breast cancer. One of them had been
treated twenty years earlier, another eight years earlier, and a third quite
recently. The women were enormously encouraging. They showed Joan
their mastectomy scars and their breast prostheses. None of them had

bothered with breast reconstruction. They begged Joan to forget about the fact that she had taken hormone replacement, pointing out that the cancer risk, while clearly increased above baseline, was still very low. They did not want her to be encumbered with useless self-blame. Cancer of the breast is just part of the risk of being a woman, just as cancer of the prostate is a man's risk. It does no good to look for blame.

Joan's friends urged her to have a second opinion at Dana-Farber. In fact, one of them had seen a Dana-Farber breast oncologist and returned to her community for care because her local oncologist, whom she liked very much, was closely affiliated with a major cancer center. The four of them enjoyed a mutual hug, and Joan called my office to start the process and get some help with the usual medical red tape. My sole contribution to her was to enable her to avoid the maze of a modern medical center. My office made her first appointment.

One week later, Joan and Bob met with Dirk Iglehart, a breast cancer surgeon and a nationally respected clinician-investigator. A Harvard Medical School graduate who had had his surgical training and all of his prior experience at Duke University Medical Center, Iglehart had recently come to Dana-Farber and the Brigham and Women's Hospital to direct breast cancer care and research in both institutions. He was one of the discoverers of the role of mutated *br*east *ca*ncer–related (BRCA) genes in the development of breast cancer in the very rare cases in which this gene plays a role.

Joan brought the mammograms and the slide of the fine-needle biopsy with her. Iglehart thought the mammograms suggested an infiltrating lobular type of breast cancer—a type that sneaks up and becomes very large before it is detected. Comparisons of all of her mammograms for two years showed the tumor progressing, but it would have been difficult to diagnose. Iglehart was quite sure that the tumor encompassed a large area of the breast and would require a complete mastectomy to remove all of it.

He told Joan and Bob that some surgeons might consider giving chemotherapy to shrink the tumor and then perform a lumpectomy, but he did not believe it would work well enough to afford her breast conservation and did not advise it. He also told Joan to forget about the possible role of hormone replacement therapy in her cancer. He agreed that there was a statistical relationship between hormones and breast cancer, but the relationship was far from linear. Joan was wise to have discontinued the hormones when she did, but estrogen replacement can also have some beneficial results. Now she should just forget about it and concentrate on the job at hand.

Iglehart laid out a plan. If Joan elected to be treated by him, he would first advise a core biopsy. The radiologist would do the procedure under ultrasound guidance in the mammography department. She would employ a much bigger needle for this biopsy. In that way, Iglehart could get a far better assessment of the invasiveness of the tumor and get all-important information about the hormone receptors that might be expressed by the tumor cells. He told Joan that breast surgeons used to explore the breast prior to mastectomy, take a piece of the tumor, and give it to the pathologist, who would do a frozen section and report on the findings during the operation. That approach had been discarded in favor of the core biopsy.

The behavior and the management of an individual's breast cancer are strongly influenced by the presence or absence of two hormone receptors. The most important of these is the estrogen receptor (ER), which is a protein that signals breast cells and breast cancer cells to multiply in the presence of the female hormones collectively called estrogens. Estrogens are produced in the ovaries and the adrenal glands and by conversion of the male sex hormone androgen to estrogen in fat cells, the adrenal glands, and the liver. If a breast cancer is ER positive—that is, it expresses the gene for the estrogen receptor protein—the growth of the tumor can be readily blocked by tamoxifen. Tamoxifen is a drug designed to sit in that receptor and prevent estrogen from getting access to it. It kills ER-positive breast cancer cells. Hence the prognosis of breast cancer is improved if it is ER positive because tamoxifen is a very effective drug. ER-positive breast cancer cells are also usually progesterone receptor (PR) positive. This information is interesting but not vital, because blockade of the estrogen receptor also shuts down the progesterone receptor gene. The PR gene depends on the activity of the ER protein for its expression.

The Her2/neu receptor is the second receptor that would be assessed by the pathologist who would receive the core biopsy. It is a receptor tyrosine kinase that stimulates growth when it interacts with a number of different growth-inducing proteins in the cancer cell. (I'll give a more detailed description of these receptors and their importance in cancer in Ken's story.) Iglehart had devoted a lot of laboratory effort to an analysis of the role of these growth factors and Her2/neu in breast cancer. Growth factors are released by many different kinds of cells in the body. Therefore, breast cancer cells are regularly bathed in such factors derived from the many supporting cells of the breast. If they express the Her2/neu receptor, the cancers will grow very rapidly.

Iglehart needed to know whether Joan's breast cancer cells were Her2/neu positive, because a recently developed monoclonal antibody called Herceptin (trastuzumab) had been developed that binds to Her2/neu and thereby blocks the capacity of growth factors to stimulate the receptor. The antibody (the first anticancer smart drug) has proven to be very useful in the management of breast cancers in which it is applicable. But since only 20 percent of breast cancers are Her2/neu positive, Iglehart did not want to spend more time discussing the receptors and the issues surrounding them until he knew whether Joan's tumor was positive or negative. He needed Joan's informed consent for the biopsy and for all of the tests for receptors that would be done on the tissue.

If Joan and Bob decided to stay with him, the biopsy would be performed in ten days under local anesthesia. Meanwhile, routine blood tests and bone scans would be scheduled to rule out any distant metastases. Joan and Bob looked at each other. They didn't need to confer. They liked Iglehart, instantly trusted him, and decided to remain at Dana-Farber for Joan's care.

# CHAPTER ELEVEN

# The Surgical Plan

A modern medical center is a maze of specialties, and even a cancer center can be likened to a rabbit warren. Every professional in a cancer center is committed to the diagnosis, treatment, and prevention of cancer and to further understanding of cancer biology. This creates a source of potential confusion for patients who need to see more than one type of specialist to complete their treatment.

The Women's Cancers Program is a perfect example of a well-intentioned but potentially confusing environment. A multidisciplinary team must manage women with breast or gynecologic cancer. In the case of breast cancer treatment, the key members of the medical team are the surgeon, the medical oncologist, and the radiation oncologist. But there are other important specialists who play vital roles. Pathologists define the extent of the tumor and document its biology. Psychologists or psychiatrists and social workers may be required to deal with severe emotional reactions. Social workers are also often needed to help patients cope with insurance issues and family crises. In addition to a large multidisciplinary staff, women with breast cancer may need very specialized facilities, including an educational resource room and a specially designed boutique to help them choose prostheses and handle chemotherapy-induced hair loss.

The forces that hold the system's feet to the fire of comprehensive care are nurse practitioners. In fact, the quality of care in most cancer centers depends on the devotion and skill of oncology nurses. Karen Pollard, an experienced nurse practitioner who works at the side of Dirk Iglehart, took over to help Joan through the maze.

Karen has felt the sting of cancer in her family. She understands the need for teamwork and makes it her business to guide patients, keeping them informed about test results and appointments for procedures. Her patients have her cell phone number. If they are anxious to know the results of a crucial test or are confused or troubled, they can reach her immediately. Karen tells me that they rarely abuse her time. When they call, it's important. The very fact that they have the number and can reach her at any time gives them peace of mind.

After the patients complete their surgical treatment and go on to medical and radiation oncology, Karen no longer runs their schedules. She turns them over to the next primary caretaker. But the patients never forget her because the surgical treatment phase is an enormous issue for many women. They need Karen desperately to help them get through an operation that may change their view of themselves forever. They respect and trust her so much that they may reach her to discuss hair loss from chemotherapy, how to deal with skin complications from chemotherapy, and other issues.

Patients are often the sources of great ideas. For example, after a mastectomy, a plastic drain is usually placed in the wound to prevent an accumulation of fluid at the base of the incision. One smart patient figured out a way to keep the drain from falling out of the wound in the shower by tying dental floss around it and winding the long end of the floss around her neck. Karen has transferred that simple idea to scores of patients.

Karen and her colleagues in nursing are indeed the force that holds it all together for the patients. The physicians may develop new approaches to treatment. Karen makes sure they are actually applied. She quickly adopted Joan's issues as her own.

The experts in the mammography division performed the core biopsy procedure under ultrasound control without a hitch. Joan actually recorded the proceedings and her subsequent discussions with her oncologists so that she could retain and sort through the barrage of new information in order to make intelligent decisions about her treatment. She commented to her nurse on the excellence of the care she received during the procedure.

The breast is a collection of milk-producing glands. A maze of ducts emerging from the glands is formed by ductal interconnections that grow in size as they approach the nipple. The whole structure is embedded in fat and held together by fibrous tissue. It is perfused by capillaries and drained by lymph channels. Cancer of the breast begins in a single epithelial cell that is in the lining of one of the mazes of ducts.

If the tumor is restricted to the duct, it is classified as stage 0 or ductal carcinoma in situ, usually shortened to DCIS. In this stage, the cancer is highly curable because it is confined to the duct. The cells have not found their way through the duct into the surrounding fat, where there are lymph channels and blood vessels into which they may pass to the draining lymph nodes under the arm or beyond into organs such as the liver, the bones, and the brain.

Though DCIS tumors remain in the duct, they may grow by traveling up and down the duct network, forming very large cancers that are still considered DCIS if they have not invaded the surrounding breast tissue. In order to invade the surrounding tissue, they must burst through the membrane and cells that form the wall of the duct. These wall-forming cells give the duct its structure. There may be important genetic changes in particular breast cancer cells that take place during the growth of DCIS—changes that enable the clone of cancer cells to penetrate the duct wall, invade the breast tissue, and become stage 1 breast cancer.

The invading cancer cells may find lymphatic channels and blood vessels in the surrounding tissue and traverse them as well. If the lump of invading cancer cells is no larger than 2 to 5 centimeters in diameter or some of the cells lodge in the draining lymph nodes in the axilla (armpit) where the lymphatics of the breast collect, the cancer is considered stage 2. If the lump is larger than 5 centimeters and has also invaded the regional nodes in the axilla, it is considered stage 3A. If it is larger than 5 centimeters or has spread to the skin, chest wall, or lymph nodes that run along the breastbone, it is considered stage 3B. Finally, if the cancer cells have disseminated widely in the blood to the organs and cancer cells are found in the bone, the liver, or the brain, the cancer is considered stage 4.

Breast cancer cells of all stages are also graded by pathologists on the basis of the state of differentiation of their nuclei. Nuclei that appear normal are called mature; very primitive-appearing nuclei are called primitive. Mature-appearing nuclei are classified as grade 1, and very primitive-appearing nuclei are classified as grade 3. Joan's cells were classified as grade 2, but neither Iglehart nor the other members of the team paid close attention to the grading system, at least at this stage of the treatment. This may be because prognosis for five-year survival is so closely associated with stage at diagnosis. Five-year survival has been the standard approach to measurement of the effects of cancer treatment.

With some exceptions, of course, five-year survival is only proportional and not equivalent to cure or disease-free survival. It is a convenient way of comparing groups of patients on different treatments, but it is a proxy figure, not always an absolute predictor. For example, five-year survival for DCIS (stage 0) is at least 97 percent. Five-year survival drops to 78 percent if regional nodes (nodes in the armpit) are involved (stage 2 or 3A) and to 23 percent if the tumor is widespread (stage 4) when it is detected. Furthermore, barely detectable tumors in the breast may be widespread at the time of diagnosis. Therefore, staging is at best a rough approximation of prognosis. But the message is simple: early detection and removal of breast cancer is the single most important weapon in managing it. That is why mammography, though admittedly very imperfect, is an important tool, and we must use it while we try to improve on it.

Iglehart went over most of the results of the core biopsy with Joan at their second meeting. (He did not have the results of the testing for estrogen receptor at that meeting.) The pathologist's diagnosis was invasive ductal carcinoma, meaning that some of the cancer cells had broken through the duct wall. Iglehart told Joan that the pathologist also described evidence of invasion into the lymph channels of the breast-supporting tissue, but he quickly added that he had no firm evidence that her armpit lymph nodes were involved. (Lymph channel invasion strongly suggests that the lymph nodes are involved.) Such a finding would place Joan's tumor at stage 2 or higher depending on its size. Iglehart admitted that axillary (armpit) lymph node involvement was possible, but he did not dwell on it.

Iglehart devoted most of his discussion of the biopsy to the behavior of the cancer cells after they had broken through the duct wall and reached the supporting tissues. They tended to form streams of replicating cells rather than a single ball. None of the streams were very dense. That is why the tumor was difficult to detect on the mammogram. The streaming behavior of the cells also implied that the overall dimensions of the cancer were probably quite large; that it would be difficult to find the margins of the tumor and therefore very hard to plan a simple lumpectomy. The appearance suggested that a mastectomy would be the best approach.

Iglehart admitted that even a mastectomy might not get out all of a streaming tumor. Joan would probably need tamoxifen therapy (if the tumor was ER positive), chemotherapy, and local radiation therapy. Without them, considerably more than half of the surgically treated patients with this type of cancer relapse. They came to an agreement on a date for surgery that would permit Joan to attend an important meeting in Washington on the national commission that supports community service curriculum development. Iglehart agreed to get the operation done early enough so that she could go to the conference even with her drain remaining in the wound. He would find her a temporary prosthesis that she could wear.

Iglehart was very reassuring to Joan: "Nobody will know that you just had surgery. You can shower; you can do anything you want. All your friends should be surprised at how well you are doing. As far as this operation is concerned, you can go home the same day. As long as the operation goes smoothly and there's no complication, the only thing you probably shouldn't do is deep-sea dive!"

Joan smiled at the thought of deep-sea diving. That wasn't quite her sport. "My friend, Janet, who's been through it, had ten of her eighteen nodes affected, and she's really good today. She told me that breast cancer isn't necessarily dire and awful. You can be strong and you can do things. That's the way I'd like to be."

Seeing that he had successfully crossed the emotional bridge from an unwise lumpectomy to the necessary mastectomy and axillary (armpit) node dissection, Iglehart pressed forward. "You'll be surprised how smoothly it will go. For instance, they'll want you to get a visiting nurse. I don't think you'll need the nurse because you'll feel much better than you expect. We do the operation under a regional anesthetic, put numbing medicine in the nerves of the ribs, and you'll be almost pain-free. Nobody is totally pain-free. And you will see patients leaving the hospital on the same day carrying their purses under their arm, on the side of their mastectomy, with their hair done and their coat on, and out the door they go."

After that airy description of the best of all possible worlds, Iglehart started to go over the potential complications. The most serious hazard is bleeding and a collection of blood at the base of the wound called a hematoma. That happens about 3 to 5 percent of the time, and it is a problem because the wound has to be reopened to drain it. The second most common complication is an infection aggravated by the plastic drain that prevents the collection of blood and fluid but connects the wound to the outside world. Patients are discharged on antibiotics to reduce that risk. Joan had not heard much about hematomas or infections as complications, but she had heard a lot about arm swelling after removal of lymph nodes from the axilla. That was the complication she wanted Iglehart to discuss.

"In the old days, when we radically removed lymph nodes and dissected them right off the big vein that goes down your arm, the chance of severe arm swelling was high due to blockage of the vein and the lymphatic channels. Nowadays, with the more limited operation under the arm, that complication should be pretty uncommon, but it still does happen, and an occasional patient will have lymphedema (arm swelling) even with the modern limited operation. I usually tell patients that there is a two to three percent chance of mild arm swelling. With exercise and massage, it's really quite controllable."

Iglehart then went on to describe the loss of sensation in the region of the mastectomy and down the arm, which would be permanent unless he could save the nerves running through the tissues that had to be removed. If he could save the nerves, they would be painful for a while as they recovered. If he had to cut them because they were in the field, Joan would be numb, but the numbness would decrease with time. He would try to save as many nerves as possible. Finally, he was sure she would recover full mobility of her arm in about two months.

Joan was disappointed, of course, that her breast cancer would require so much surgical treatment. Fortunately, the initial X-rays had already shown that she was not an obvious stage 4, but she knew enough about breast cancer to accept the fact that it can be widespread without leaving any traces in the early stages. Iglehart had already mentioned chemotherapy as an adjunct for the surgical treatment. If her nodes were positive, she would certainly get chemotherapy and radiation therapy as well. She agreed to the mastectomy and hoped for the best. Iglehart concluded the discussion by telling Joan that he would keep her informed about the special tests that were performed on the biopsy to determine whether her cancer cells expressed estrogen and Her2/neu receptors. These pathology reports would be ready in a few days.

Almost as an afterthought, Joan took up the question of breast reconstruction only to reemphasize to Iglehart that she was not interested. Her discussions with Janet and her other friends with cancer had helped her to make up her mind.

Joan explained to Iglehart, "I remember Janet saying, 'Oh, it's an appendage. Just think of it as an appendage. You don't need it, anyway.' That's helped me to think of it as something I can do without. I don't want to go through reconstruction." Iglehart totally agreed, and they left their discussion at that point.

While Joan's impending mastectomy should strike us as a serious operation, it is a much smaller surgery than a woman with any kind of breast cancer would have anticipated forty years ago. William Halsted, the master of surgery at Johns Hopkins, had pioneered the radical mastectomy in the final decade of the nineteenth century. Although revered as the father of modern surgery, Halsted experimented with cocaine as an anesthetic and became addicted. He held strong opinions, and his pronouncements influenced generations of surgeons. The Halsted radical mastectomy was the only acceptable surgical procedure for breast cancer when I began my career in hematology and oncology in the mid-1950s at the National Cancer Institute. Why did it vanish?

Shortly after Joan's conference with Iglehart, I asked him about the events that led breast surgeons to abandon the radical mastectomy. Iglehart explained that Halsted simply did not understand the biology of the disease. Halsted thought the tumor arose in the breast and moved stepwise from the breast to the draining lymph nodes, then to other organs such as the skin, liver, bones, and brain. Hence he designed a very mutilating and often disabling operation that removed the breast, the muscles under it, and all the lymph nodes in the armpit. But breast cancer simply does not spread stepwise.

Depending on the genetic abnormalities of the tumor, it may be very stable in the breast or it may spread rapidly and widely, very early, sometimes stopping in the nodes of the armpit but sometimes spreading throughout the body. The massive, often crippling, and completely unnecessary Halsted operation does nothing to change those facts. Yet the procedure was the established approach to breast cancer until the 1970s because Halsted was one of the fathers of American surgery. His reputation was Jovian and there were no competing hypotheses. Furthermore, the surgical cure rates achieved by Halsted's operation were impressive—80 percent in lymph node–negative breast cancer and 30 to 40 percent in lymph node–positive cases. That is about the same as the surgical cure rates today, but today we achieve these rates with far less mutilating surgery. (Other modalities of treatment have vastly improved the cure rates for lymph node–positive cases.)

Iglehart admitted that the Halsted operation only died in the 1970s because women began to reject it. They spurned older surgeons who favored the operation and turned to younger ones who were willing to do lumpectomies or simple mastectomies. Within two years, during Iglehart's residency at Duke, the Halsted operation disappeared even though the clinical trials instigated by questioning surgeons like George Crile, Umberto Veronesi, and Bernard Fisher—who proved that far less invasive surgery was just as effective—were not completed until several years later.

Other radical operations were also in vogue in the 1950s and into the 1980s. In 1896, George Beatson, a Scottish surgeon, reported regression of breast cancer in two patients who had had their ovaries removed. A half century later, Charles Huggins and David Bergenstal at the University of Chicago showed that adrenalectomy (removal of the adrenal glands atop the kidneys) would reduce the growth of human breast cancer. Huggins received the Nobel Prize in 1966 for his work on the relationship of hormones to the growth of breast and prostate cancer. (We now know that the male hormone, androgen, is converted to estrogen in the adrenal gland as well as in the liver and in fat cells by an enzyme called aromatase. Today, we have a drug that effectively blocks aromatase—adrenalectomy is no longer even considered in breast cancer.) During my brief experience at NCI, I saw many women undergo removal of the ovaries, the adrenals, and even the pituitary gland in the brain in a vain effort to control their metastatic breast cancer. Those procedures (other than removal of the ovaries for rare cases with inherited susceptibility to breast and ovarian cancer) have largely disappeared as well.

Iglehart went on to remind me that the so-called epidemic of breast cancer that has been observed in the past twenty years is largely due to a proliferation of postmenopausal ER-positive cases. These are cases that tend to respond well to estrogen blockade with drugs like tamoxifen and aromatase inhibition as well as to low-invasive surgery, radiation therapy, and chemotherapy. The ER-negative cases are more resistant to treatment and do not fare as well. "By the way," he said, "I just learned that Joan's tumor is ER positive and (as expected) Her2/neu negative." I was glad to hear that news. Joan's tumor might be large, but it had favorable receptors.

Iglehart told me that he had advised Joan to have a mastectomy because he did not believe that he could remove her tumor with a lumpectomy that would leave very much if any breast and still encompass all of the tumor. He was glad that Joan had rejected breast reconstruction surgery because he thought it should be prescribed carefully and sparingly. For some women, it blunts the psychological effect of mastectomy, but it can be a very difficult operation.

The breast cancer surgery field has matured to the point where we know its limits. The goal of surgery is to remove all the gross local disease and gain diagnostic information to inform the next step of therapy. The surgeon must achieve normal tissue margins around the tumor and determine whether armpit lymph nodes are involved. That is the information to be passed on to the radiotherapist and the medical oncologist who will take over when the surgeon has completed his or her task. By 1990, half the patients in the United States (or at least in major academic centers where these details were documented) were treated with lumpectomy and radiation with some degree of breast conservation, and half were managed with mastectomies. Of those who had mastectomies, probably a third to a half had reconstruction.

I asked for more details about postmastectomy breast reconstruction, though I knew that Iglehart is not enthusiastic about the procedure. His response was at best lukewarm. I pointed out that radiation would damage all the vessels in the area of the reconstruction, and Iglehart agreed.

"You can do a saline or silicone implant after radiation, but the results can be really bad; patients may get a tremendous amount of fibrosis and get a little tennis ball on the chest instead of a soft tissue mound. So you're forced to bring in healthy tissue from the periphery using muscles that have not been irradiated to provide a blood supply for the fat pad taken with the muscle. These are huge operations that are called TRAM flaps. I think women need to be warned that this is a vast amount of surgery. I want our people to be very critical of the operation. We can do it and do it very well, but we shouldn't push it. If you've ever seen a TRAM flap, you would know what I mean and what an undertaking it is. I just think patients need to be fully informed before they rush into it."

I asked Iglehart about the dissection of nodes in the armpit. I wanted to know how he collaborates with the radiotherapists to avoid radiation therapy in a surgically disturbed area and whether he is beginning to adopt sentinel node biopsy instead of dissection in the armpit. Would Joan have a dissection or a sentinel node biopsy? What was her risk of arm edema?

Iglehart told me that sentinel lymph node biopsy has replaced armpit lymph node dissection for many patients. Rather than removing fifteen or twenty lymph nodes in every patient, surgeons just remove one to three lymph nodes that are the most likely to contain metastasis. These are the sentinel nodes. They choose the nodes for removal by injecting either a dye or a radioactive tracer into the tumor and waiting for a period of time, usually less than an hour, until there's been uptake of radioactivity or blue dye in the lymph nodes. Then they make a small incision in the armpit and find the radioactive or the blue lymph nodes. These lymph nodes would probably receive the cancer cells first.

If sentinel nodes are negative, then with probably 90 to 95 percent assurance, the rest of the lymph nodes will be negative. Further dissection will be unrevealing. If a sentinel node is positive for metastasis, then there is probably a 40 or 50 percent chance that other lymph nodes in the armpit will be positive. In such a patient, it is advisable to perform a complete dissection to determine the fraction of affected nodes. If the majority of nodes are positive, Eric Winer, the chief of breast medical oncology at Dana-Farber, would assume that the disease is widespread and would add an additional chemotherapeutic drug to the patient's treatment regimen. Jay Harris, the radiation oncologist, who edited a classic book on breast diseases, explains that he needs an enumeration of positive lymph nodes to plan his radiation portals. If a sentinel is the only positive node, however, he wouldn't radiate the rest of the nodes in the armpit, and Winer would not add the additional chemotherapy.

In Joan's case, Iglehart was quite certain that several nodes would be positive because her tumor was large and had a streaming appearance. Therefore, he planned a node dissection without a sentinel node test. He was confident that her risk of arm swelling would be low if the radiotherapists avoided the surgical field. He was certain that Eric Winer would recommend both estrogen receptor blockade with tamoxifen and full combination chemotherapy.

Iglehart then touched upon an aspect of medical care that has been troubling to physicians and patients alike. Gone are the days when physicians dictated treatment to patients. This is particularly the case when male physicians care for female patients. The domineering relationship of physician to patient has been replaced with a cornucopia of options, and the burden has fallen on patients to make the final decisions. This has created a new stress—the tension caused by overinformation, much of which is unreliable.

Iglehart wanted Joan to have a mastectomy and a node dissection (now called a modified radical mastectomy). He wanted her to have radiation to the armpit and take the risk of arm swelling, and he wanted her to have full combination chemotherapy and hormone blockade because he was quite certain that the totality of such combined treatment would give her a 70 to 80 percent chance of disease-free survival. But Iglehart knew that he must make those recommendations without commandeering Joan's right to make her own decisions. Fortunately, Joan is a down-to-earth woman who does not fly toward extreme positions. And Joan has a very supportive family and a bevy of good friends, several of whom have traveled the breast cancer road. In that setting, she came to her own decision and agreed with Iglehart. But she might have rejected chemotherapy or hormone blockade, or she might have insisted on a double mastectomy to avoid the risk, however small, of a recurrence in the opposite breast. She did neither, and Iglehart planned the surgery after introducing her to Winer and Harris, who would take over when the surgical phase of treatment had been completed.

Thus, Joan was launched on what is now considered standard care for metastatic estrogen receptor–positive breast cancer—a process that would require a five-year commitment and more than a little discomfort but would produce a high likelihood of success. But are there future treatments that could assure an even higher success rate?

From the surgeon's point of view, there are two main pathways of discovery that make a difference in outcome: better control of estrogen influence on estrogen receptor–positive tumors by aromatase inhibitors (drugs that prevent the conversion of androgen to estrogen in the adrenal glands, the liver, and fat cells) and the development of smart drugs to inhibit growth-stimulating receptors in addition to Her2/neu, the receptor that is driven by epidermal growth factor. The Her2/neu receptor is active in only 20 percent of breast cancers, and, until very recently, the only weapon against it was a monoclonal antibody. We have to find the drivers of the other 80 percent and find the smart drugs that will shut them down.

Iglehart is particularly fascinated by the collaborative work of the Netherlands Cancer Institute with Stephen Friend and his former colleagues at Rosetta Impharmatics (now owned by Merck). They clearly demonstrated that the prognosis of breast cancer and, more recently, lung cancer can be related to the measurement of the expression of thousands of genes in the tumor with the special method called microarray analysis used by Scott Armstrong and Todd Golub for MLL leukemia. This should lead to new targets for drugs because high expression of a gene by a cancer suggests that the cancer relies on that gene for its survival.

"Cancer research," Iglehart concluded, "is becoming systems research. Whether we measure gene expression or the proteins that are produced or look for gene mutations directly, we are beginning to look at very large numbers of molecules simultaneously and obtain a global view of a cancer. Much of our work is based on information technology that we never used before. Of course, that will inexorably force us to look more systematically at the other major part of the equation, which is the patient herself. We are just now beginning to examine the tumor, but we have to keep in mind that the capacity of the tumor to grow is also influenced by patient age, ethnicity, and genetic background. Host genes play a very important role in the maintenance of a tumor."

That remark reminded me of a wonderful review of tumor–host relationships published in 2000 by two leading cancer researchers, Douglas Hanahan, of the University of California in San Francisco, and Robert Weinberg, of Massachusetts Institute of Technology. They emphasize that cancer is an organ growing in a host. The host has to provide a permissive environment or the cancer cannot develop. In 2005, Nellie Polyak, of Dana-Farber, devised a unique method to perform a massive systems analysis of gene chemistry in the *normal* cells surrounding an incipient breast cancer. She found subtle changes, known as epigenetic changes, in some of the thousands of normal genes. Her findings provide strong evidence that Hanahan and Weinberg are exactly right. The normal breast cells of many women actually foster the growth of a cancer by turning some of their genes on and others off in such a way as to enhance tumor cell growth.

In very rare cases (less than 5 percent of breast cancer patients), women inherit loss-of-function mutations in genes that repair DNA after inevitable damage by mutating chemicals or solar radiation. These genes are called antioncogenes because they prevent the onset of cancer. If just one gene is mutated and inherited, nothing happens. But there is a high likelihood that within a few decades the defective gene will be *copied* in at least one cell of a breast or an ovary. Then both genes in that cell will be abnormal. The untoward event will render the cell incapable of DNA repair, and breast cancer and/or ovarian cancer will be the result. Mutations in these antioncogenes (called breast cancer–associated or BRCA genes) are responsible for familial breast or ovarian cancer.

Other examples of mutations in important antioncogenes include the sniffing proteins described in Mario's story. Such proteins—for example, p53—are responsible for detecting breaks and errors in genes within DNA and consigning such cells to the death pathway. In the absence of their function, cancer may well occur. In fact, p53 deficiency is a very frequent acquired defect in many common sporadic cancers. In addition, there is a very rare form of familial cancer called Li-Fraumeni syndrome that is characterized by an extremely high incidence at a young age of leukemia, sarcomas, and breast cancer. It is caused by an inherited abnormality of p53. In such rare families, one of the pair of chromosome 17s has a defective or absent p53 gene. Family members who inherit that chromosome have a high likelihood of copying it in a breast duct, bone, or blood-forming cell. That bad cell now has two defective p53 genes, and breast cancer, bone cancer, brain tumors, leukemia, and other cancers may result.

I came away from my discussion with Iglehart confident that Joan was in the right hands. He has the technical expertise and a broad understanding of the biology of breast cancer. He is a master at building teams that will solve problems in a collaborative manner. He would get Joan started on her road back to health, make sure that his colleagues in medical and radiation oncology finish the job, and keep all of us working on new approaches that would be ready for Joan should she need them in the future.

In a few days, Joan entered the hospital. Iglehart held her hand as the anesthesiologists gave her a regional block of the nerves of her left chest and a mild sedative to make her drowsy. As she was wheeled into the operating room and the skin of her left chest was sterilized with solutions of iodine and alcohol, she recited a prayer that one of her friends who had had breast cancer very recently had advised her to say:

> May the light of God surround me
> May the love of God enfold me
> May the power of God protect me
> May the presence of God watch over me
> For wherever I am, God is.

The modified radical mastectomy and axillary node dissection took less than two hours. Joan was soon in the recovery area and rapidly transferred from there to her hospital room with a drain at the base of the wound to rid it of blood and fluids. She was very tired and there was some discomfort. She wanted to sleep. Iglehart decided to hold her overnight and sent her home with Bob the next day to await the results of the pathology. Then the next stage of planning would be presented to her and her family.

Well before the scheduled conference with Joan and her family, Iglehart received the report from his colleagues in pathology. The tumor was big. It measured at least 6.5 centimeters in diameter. It was largely confined to breast ducts, but it also streamed across the ducts into supporting tissue. It definitely invaded the lymphatic channels of the breast. There were excellent margins of normal tissue around the streaming tumor cells. The nuclei of the cancer cells were classified as grade 2. Six of the eleven dissected lymph nodes were positive for cancer cells. The cancer cells were estrogen receptor positive and Her2/neu negative. In summary, Joan had stage 3A, grade 2 ER-positive Her2/neu-negative postmenopausal breast cancer, the type of cancer commonly seen in the past two decades.

Iglehart had suspected that Joan would require much more treatment and had already prepared her for that when they had met to discuss the operation. Now he was certain. In her present state, her chances of relapse without further treatment were well in excess of 50 percent, probably close to 70 percent. In women like her, more than half of the relapses would occur within five years. That is what I saw following the Halsted radical mastectomy for lymph node–positive breast cancer in the 1950s. Iglehart was confident that Joan's risk of relapse could be substantially reduced. It was fair to say that the last fifty years of progress in breast cancer would cut her risk of relapse from close to 70 percent to near 20 percent—not a perfect answer by any means but a huge improvement over the days when the best surgeons were disfiguring and damaging the arms of women and watching so many of them relapse.

Joan would hear the results of her surgery in her next two meetings, the first with Iglehart and the second with Eric Winer. These two meetings would be followed by a conference with Jay Harris to plan her radiation therapy.

# CHAPTER TWELVE

# The Medical Plan

B efore Joan met with Jay Harris and Eric Winer, I had a discussion with Winer so that I could be prepared to answer any questions that Joan might ask me without creating confusion. I had recruited Winer, a highly experienced breast oncologist, from Duke to run the medical oncology section of the breast program within the Women's Cancers Program at Dana-Farber and the Brigham and Women's Hospital. Eric is a brilliant physician with warmth that is noticeable as soon as he enters the room. Since childhood, he has dealt with his own lifelong bout with chronic illness and the complications of therapy. No one understands better than Eric what it is to face a serious long-term illness, and he knows that therapy can have real and unsuspected side effects. Yet he remains undaunted, follows a punishing schedule without complaint, and even rides a bicycle to raise money for cancer research. In 2003, Eric and several others bicycled across the country with Lance Armstrong to improve public awareness of cancer treatment. Eric cannot be defeated.

In the early to mid-1960s at the National Cancer Institute (NCI), Frei and Freireich were making progress in combination chemotherapy for childhood leukemia as described in Mario's story. Later in the 1960s, Vincent DeVita and his colleagues in the NCI Medicine Branch used combination chemotherapy with success in the management of Hodgkin's disease and began to make inroads on the treatment of other lymphomas.

The initial combination for Hodgkin's disease was a four-drug regimen that included the first anticancer drug, an alkylating agent called nitrogen mustard (mechloethamine). Alkylating agents work somewhat like radiation. They diffusely damage DNA by forcing chemical bonds between molecules that are not normally bound together. This effect is called cross-linking. An intravenous alkylating agent may find cancer cells anywhere in the body and cross-link their DNA enough to alert the sniffing proteins like p53 to send them down the death pathway. The second drug was vincristine (Oncovin), which is described in Mario's story. The third was a second alkylating agent called procarbazine, and prednisone was the fourth drug. The acronym for the combination was MOPP, and it worked well.

A decade later, another group of collaborators reported their successful approach to the non-Hodgkin's lymphomas with a new combination that grouped the orally active alkylating agent cyclophosphamide (Cytoxan) with hydroxydaunomycin (Adriamycin), Oncovin, and prednisone. The acronym for this brew was CHOP.

Thus, the hematological malignancies were beginning to give way to combination chemotherapy, but there was no apparent progress in the common solid tumors like breast cancer. NCI officialdom, under pressure from patient groups and Congress to make headway in the common malignancies, requested the Medicine Branch to begin trials in breast cancer. Accordingly, in the early 1970s, George Canellos and his colleagues reported that the combination of Cytoxan, melphalan (another orally active alkylating agent), and a methotrexate-like inhibitor of folate reductase called 5-fluorouracil was active in metastatic breast cancer.

Now came the big question. Would this combination, known as CMF, be useful if given directly after mastectomy (so-called adjuvant therapy) and delay or even prevent recurrence? This was critical because the argument about the pathophysiology of breast cancer was not resolved at that time. Halsted had proposed that the disease spreads locally from the breast. Others held that the disease is often widespread at the outset. If the latter were true, a burst of adjuvant chemotherapy that was known to be active against the cancer cells should delay or even abort recurrence.

To settle the argument, NCI gave a contract to Gianni Bonadonna and his colleagues in Milan, Italy, who gave CMF as adjuvant treatment to 207 women with axillary (armpit) lymph node–positive breast cancer directly after the Halsted radical mastectomy. A group of 179 women who received only the standard surgery served as controls. The results, published in 1976, were striking. After twenty-seven months of follow-up, 24 percent of the control patients had relapsed (many in distant sites) while only 5 percent of the CMF-treated patients had relapsed. There was now no question that breast cancer is a widespread disease and adjuvant chemotherapy can delay or even prevent relapse. The results additionally supported the growing view of surgeons that less surgery and more active adjuvant therapy provided the path to progress in breast cancer. The fundamental conflict was settled. The practical issue would be the search for more and more effective drugs.

Beginning in the early 1980s, similar trials showed that combinations containing anthracyclines such as Adriamycin and taxanes (inhibitors of cell division originally derived from yew trees) were thought to be superior to and were certainly more convenient than those with melphalan and 5-fluorouracil. Therefore, CMF was gradually changed to CA with or without the addition of T (for Taxol), the latter depending on the extent of lymph node involvement. Currently, combination chemotherapy can be expected to reduce the relative risk of relapse by about 20 percent. That translates to an important contribution for an individual like Joan with nearly a 70 percent risk of relapse, but much more is needed. Fortunately for Joan, the administration of hormone receptor blockade with tamoxifen to an ER-positive tumor produces another 40 to 50 percent of relative risk reduction. Radiation therapy probably offers yet another 10 percent. So a plan could be made for Joan that would give her a 60 to 70 percent relative risk reduction, which would bring her absolute risk of relapse down to close to 20 percent.

Of course, the first question I asked Winer was whether a four-drug combination would offer a higher relative risk reduction than three, and if a five-drug combination would be better than four. That was the case in acute lymphoblastic leukemia treatment, in which a six-drug combination proved to be the most beneficial.

Winer was cautious. He first emphasized that unlike the situation in the leukemias, we are currently unable to select the patients who might be better candidates for chemotherapy, except that ER-negative and Her2/neu-positive tumors tended to be more aggressive and more responsive to chemotherapy. (Indeed, in 2006, the National Cancer Institute announced a clinical trial designed to determine whether some women with estrogen receptor–positive breast cancer required chemotherapy at all.)

Winer agreed that the studies carried out in the 1970s clearly demonstrated the value of three-drug combinations over single agents, though

CAT, the most recent combination of three drugs, can be given sequentially with equal results. I asked him whether he would consider a trial with five drugs instead of three.

"It wouldn't be out of the question. The real challenge would be to design the trial in such a way as to determine the piece of the new combination that was really important so that we didn't waste toxicity and compromise doses of active agents by adding in something that wasn't working particularly well."

Winer described recent trials of CAT in which the cyclophosphamide (Cytoxan) dose was doubled and quadrupled. The results were unimpressive. Similarly unimpressive results were obtained when the dose of Adriamycin was increased. So we are at the right doses with the drugs we currently use, but we really do not know whether the addition of more drugs would be beneficial. For example, one might consider the addition of melphalan and 5-fluorouracil to the CAT regimen because they are known to be active. But the toxicity would be serious. It could only be ethically offered to women at very high risk of relapse such as those who are ER negative and cannot benefit from tamoxifen.

Winer reminded me that a trial was now in progress to test alteration of the schedule of the three-drug CAT regimen. The theory is that if the doses are given with narrower time intervals, there might be a small but very real improvement in results. Joan would start her treatment before the results of that trial would be known. (Later the trial proved positive—there is a small benefit to interval reduction.)

We went on to discuss the brief and highly contentious interest in the use of massive doses of drugs—doses sufficient to destroy the bone marrow—followed by infusion of bone marrow cells that had been obtained and frozen prior to the drug dosing. These so called auto-marrow transplants became widely if briefly accepted in the 1990s before they were found to add little or nothing to the outcome of the disease. But desperate patients demanded the treatment, and physicians in many centers believed they had to offer it to maintain their referrals. Some of us still wonder whether the approach might not make sense. However, the opportunity to do clinical trials vanished in the very brief period when the procedure was approved for general use. Now it is largely forgotten. Is there something of value in that concept?

Winer thought about the subject carefully, reviewed the history, and concluded, "I don't see a lot of interest in pursuing this further, although

I do believe that if we had the answers ten years ago that we have today, we might then have started a series of trials trying to define which group of women might benefit from this very high-dose therapy. But breast cancer just doesn't seem to be a disease that, generally speaking, is sensitive to dose escalation beyond a certain level."

Winer agrees with Iglehart that blockade of growth factor receptors by smart drugs offers a much more promising approach to breast cancer than does DNA damage to the tumor (and normal tissues) through carpet-bombing chemotherapy. The excellent response of ER-positive patients to tamoxifen and to aromatase inhibitors and the response of Her2/neu-positive patients to Herceptin are his examples.

A very recent study of sequential tamoxifen and an aromatase inhibitor has shown an additive effect of the combination. Blockade of Her2/neu by Herceptin has been evaluated in the adjuvant setting in the United States and abroad. (The antibody is given at the onset of initial treatment to a patient with Her2/neu-positive breast cancer.) Joan would not have qualified for those studies because her cancer is Her2/neu negative, but the results of the study have already shown a 50 percent improvement in disease-free survival in the Her2/neu-positive patients who received the antibody. That is a major advance in therapy and shows once again how important it is to bring up all the guns immediately in the treatment of cancer.

There is a real need for much more basic and clinical research in the growth factor area, particularly for ER-negative tumors. As Winer emphasized, "The hope is, of course, that we are going to have many more Herceptins, some of which may be used together."

The problem we currently face is that we do not yet have more Herceptins. The search for additional tyrosine kinase receptors or other growth factor receptors or signaling molecules in breast cancer is taking place in many laboratories and companies. Recent reports from the Sanger Laboratory at Cambridge University suggest that oncogenic kinase mutations other than Her2/neu are uncommon in breast cancer.

The conversation with Eric was helpful. I looked forward to hearing from Joan after she met with him and with Iglehart for their planning conference.

# CHAPTER THIRTEEN

# The Baton Is Passed

I glehart was good to his word. Joan's strength returned very rapidly, and she was ready for action when she returned with her daughter, Ellen, to see him for her first postoperative visit. She was already planning her promised trip to Washington for the national meeting that she wanted to attend. In fact, her first question was about the drain and air travel. Would she risk a fluid accumulation at the base of the wound if she traveled? Iglehart looked at the wound and actually pulled the drain out, pronouncing her ready for travel.

Then the harder part of the discussion started. Iglehart gave Joan the results of the surgery and told her that six of the eleven lymph nodes were positive. For a few seconds, Joan didn't hear him. She wanted things to be simple, and simplicity was not in the cards. Just as Bob had not heard her when she told him she had breast cancer, she did not immediately hear Iglehart when he told her that she had stage 3A breast cancer and would require triple chemotherapy and radiation therapy to boot. She began to recover her hearing while he was explaining the relative risk reductions provided by tamoxifen, CA(T) chemotherapy, and radiation. Iglehart broke off and asked her how she was feeling. Joan thought he was inquiring about her postoperative symptoms, not her present feelings. "David Nathan called me Sunday night, and he said I might get the postop blahs on Monday and Tuesday, and I felt a little bit of blahs yesterday."

Iglehart interrupted to tell her that her blahs of yesterday were not the point. First of all, he boasted, her operation was perfect and his patients don't get postop blahs. "Do you know when people get the blahs after all this? People get the blahs at the very end. Two weeks after you've finished your radiation therapy and we say, 'See you in six months,' that's when people get the blahs. During the period of time that you're under our care and receiving therapy, there's so much going on that you won't have time for the blahs. You'll feel good because you're being treated, and then at the end you think, 'Gosh, now it's all done.' That may make you begin to worry about the future. As you know, this is something that you have to live with and live around. It's not going to go away. At no point will somebody say, 'Okay, you're done. You're cured.' It's not like a gallbladder operation. The fear is going to be there, and that's just going to become part of your life. And you just have to not let it get the best of you. I am certain that you will deal with all of this and we will help you."

Then he suddenly changed the subject and the two talked animatedly about Joan's trip to Washington and the role of community service learning in the K–12 school experience. Obviously, Iglehart saw this conversation as an important way to focus Joan on real life through the tough year of hormone blockade and chemo and radiation therapy and the year it would take to recover. Though the discussion might have seemed irrelevant to an outsider, it was Iglehart's way of letting Joan know that he was vitally interested in her as a person. He knew that would help her refocus on herself rather than her cancer and would be very valuable if an untoward event occurred in the future because it would help her bond to him as her caretaker.

Then Iglehart turned the conversation back to the next steps. He would schedule Joan for a bone scan and a CT scan of the chest to be sure that there was no evidence of breast cancer metastatic to the skeleton or the lungs. He would also schedule appointments for Joan first with Winer, the medical oncologist, and then with Jay Harris, the radiation oncologist. He told Joan that he was quite confident there would be no fluid accumulation in her wound and emphasized that he could easily be reached if she needed him.

As she was preparing to leave, Joan mentioned that her mother died in her early seventies of ovarian cancer. There were cases of breast cancer in the family and other cancers as well. Was she at risk? What about her ovaries? Would it make sense to remove them? Was her daughter at risk?

Iglehart listened carefully. "Yes, it does make some sense [to remove your ovaries] even though there is a vanishingly small chance that you have a mutated BRCA gene." He didn't dismiss the history, but he thought it was unconvincing. He or Winer would be willing to do the tests for the known BRCA gene defects, but normal tests would not exclude some presently unknown cancer susceptibility gene. Removal of Joan's ovaries at some point would reduce her risk of ovarian cancer to zero. Joan thought for a moment and said that she would talk it over with her family.

Almost as an afterthought while pulling on her coat, Joan mentioned that she is a great believer in alternative healing programs including meditation and nutritional supplements. Iglehart had heard that opinion many times and only asked her to be sure to tell Winer about the details of any programs she pursued, particularly any drugs or supplements that might compromise her cancer therapy. She readily agreed. She went home to plan her trip to Washington, confirm her scheduled CT and bone scans, and schedule her appointment with Winer.

A week later, Joan, accompanied by Bob, returned to the Women's Cancers Program to see Winer and meet his younger associate, Ann Partridge. Joan listened attentively to Winer. She knew Winer was an expert in breast oncology—indeed, one of the leaders in the field. But she was immediately attracted to Partridge. There was a near-chemical bond between the two women as soon as they met. From that moment, Joan wanted Partridge to be her doctor, and Winer was wise enough to encourage the relationship. But before he handed the baton that had been given to him by Iglehart over to Partridge, he outlined the next few months of Joan's care.

Winer began with a general statement about the development of the plan. He pointed out that patients often think they are listening and absorbing all the details when they are not. He was quite sure that Joan would go back to her home and realize that there were wide gaps in her understanding. He urged her to call him or Partridge with those questions and get them resolved. Then he went over some of the ground that had been covered by Iglehart, emphasizing that Joan and her family would have to develop a new way of looking at illness. We are all accustomed to having an illness and getting over it. In the case of breast cancer, patients can never tell themselves that they have it totally behind them. True, as time goes on, there is less and less of a chance of recurrence, but the risk never falls to zero. So Joan and those who love her would have to adopt a tough-minded approach that emphasizes savoring every day and always looking forward to the next one.

Winer then talked about the benefits and downsides of tamoxifen and chemotherapy, pointing out that tamoxifen is far less toxic than chemotherapy and is the most beneficial of Joan's proposed therapies, but it must be given for five years. Chemotherapy is unpleasant, but it is delivered over a much shorter period—about six months. Radiation therapy follows chemotherapy. It is annoying because it must be given daily for five days a week over several weeks, but it is usually well tolerated. The total package would bring her risk of relapse during her lifetime down from her present near-70 percent to close to 20 percent. And every year of disease-free survival would lower her overall risk.

The plan would be completed after the results were known of the CT and bone scans scheduled for that day. Eric promised to call Joan as soon as he knew the results. It would be a long day of waiting to get the tests done, but Joan and Bob had Tootsie Rolls, water, pretzels, and a couple of good books. They were prepared to hunker down and wait. Joan's only voiced concern was to get through it all in time for a trip to Tibet the following summer.

Then Winer began to describe the side effects of the proposed chemotherapy, including reversible hair loss and nausea and vomiting in about half the patients, which is well controlled with antinausea medication in almost all the patients. Joan's white blood cells would be lower during the treatment, making her susceptible to infections from the germs on and in her own body. There was much less infection risk from the germs of others. She could go to church, movies, and meetings without risk. But she would have to report symptoms such as high fever or severe lethargy, and it would be important to keep her primary physician in her home city in the loop of information so that her doctor could manage any emergency that might arise.

Joan and Bob understood Winer completely because they had heard most of the information already from Iglehart. But they appreciated the repetition. There was a lot of information to absorb, and the fact processing was slowed by their anxiety. They needed to hear the plan several times before they could incorporate it completely.

Joan had two further points that she wanted to discuss. She had decided to forgo the opportunity to have genetic testing for the two known BRCA genes. She was concerned about the possibility that she might have inherited such a gene from her mother, but the fact that a negative test would not rule out a familial susceptibility persuaded Joan to reject the test. Winer agreed with her reasoning completely. Joan also decided that at the end of her chemo and radiation treatment and after she had completely recovered, she would have her ovaries removed. Winer agreed wholeheartedly with that notion as well. (Joan had a complete hysterectomy including removal of her ovaries a year after she completed the nontamoxifen components of her treatment.)

Joan concluded her meeting with Winer and Partridge with the question about alternative and holistic healing that she had raised with Iglehart. She wanted to know whether Winer approved of her plan to visit a physician near her home who prescribed diets and food supplements that were purported to strengthen the immune system and thereby defeat cancer. And she wanted to purchase some relaxation tapes marketed at the nearby Beth Israel Deaconess Medical Center.

Winer was certain that relaxation tapes could do no harm and they might be very useful. He avoided comment on the unhappy fact that Americans spend billions of dollars on totally untested and unregulated treatments, many of which are actually prescribed by licensed physicians and sold by their offices. He said nothing negative about the issues associated with the delivery of prayer therapy by physicians. Winer was wise enough to stay away from the controversies and remain supportive.

"I tend to separate what I call the complementary therapies into two groups: things you put into your body and things that you do to your head and body. It's very hard for me to imagine that things like meditation, relaxation techniques, and prayer for some people could possibly do physical harm to patients, and it's easy to imagine that they could do some good. I have to be more careful about diet and food supplements because I can imagine that massive diet changes or supplements could affect chemo- and even radiation therapy, and they could possibly interfere with estrogen blockade. In fact, some food additives have estrogens in them. So I am wary about these untested diets and food supplements."

Winer pointed out that Dana-Farber has a substantial complementary therapy program and that he would be happy to link Joan to the nurses who direct it. In that way, she could pursue her interest and remain safe. Joan and Bob were pleased. Winer agreed to call them to start treatment as soon as the scan results were known. They marched off to the radiology department for the imaging studies. Then they went home to await the call that would launch the treatment plan under the hands-on direction of Partridge, with Winer hovering in the background.

# CHAPTER FOURTEEN

# The Consequences of Therapy

As predicted, Joan's CT scan of the chest and bone scan were completely normal. Winer called her with that good news and asked her to schedule her first treatment with intravenous Adriamycin and Cytoxan in the Dana-Farber ambulatory therapy center. Adriamycin, an anthracycline, binds to DNA and prevents its repair. Cytoxan is an alkylating agent that cross-links DNA. Joan accepted her treatment plan readily, albeit fearfully, but she told Winer that she hoped she would not be asked to take Taxol, the cousin of vincristine. It is a strong inhibitor of cell division. Her friend, Janet, had taken Taxol. It is damaging to peripheral nerves, and Janet had pain in the bottoms of her feet and uncertain gait for years after taking the drug. Winer ducked the question for the moment. He felt that Partridge would soon gain Joan's confidence, and the two of them would reach an agreement about Taxol. He knew that Joan would need Taxol to lower her risk of relapse.

It is very important for patients with a serious long-term disease to retain some control over their medical agenda. A paternalistic approach by a physician—an "I know best" attitude—is often counterproductive. One of the most valuable aspects of complementary therapy is that it empowers patients to participate actively in their treatment instead of feeling like hopeless victims suspended at the end of a needle connected to an intravenous drip of toxic medicine. So Winer realized at once that Joan would have to work her way slowly to the Taxol part of the treatment. And there was no rush.

Partridge and Winer had decided to do a trial in which Taxol would be given during radiation therapy in order to save patients a lot of time.

The combined radiation and Taxol treatment would not start for four months. The first order of business was to get Joan started on Adriamycin and Cytoxan. Joan's DNA was about to get a nasty bludgeoning. She began her first treatment in the October that followed the summer of her surgery.

Both Adriamycin and Cytoxan damage DNA; cells with such damage are detected by sniffing proteins. The phagocytic (or "eating cells") that line the tissues then swallow the DNA-damaged cells. But the drugs are entirely nonselective. All of the cells of the body that can be reached by the drug are poisoned. Cancer cells are, however, particularly vulnerable because their chromosomes and hence their genes are already in disarray as a result of the disease process itself. The added stress of the drug effects tips the effete cancer cells over the edge into the death pathway. Normal cells with intact chromosomes are more resistant. But the resistance of normal cells is relative. Many of them, particularly those that divide rapidly—such as the cells that produce hair, the skin cells, the lining or epithelial cells of the stomach and intestines, the lining cells of the bladder, and the vital cells of the blood that carry oxygen, fight infection, and clot the blood—are badly damaged.

Four treatments with Cytoxan and Adriamycin every two and a half to three weeks will cause hair loss and lowering of the white blood cell count with the risk of infection. There is also the risk of nausea, mouth sores, inflammation and bleeding in the bladder (particularly with Cytoxan), and anemia. But that's not all. The intravenous treatment produces a very high drug level for a short time—enough to allow the toxic drug access to the centers in the brain and the peripheral receptors that trigger vomiting. Fortunately, the pharmaceutical industry has responded by making drugs called antiemetics to block the signals in the nervous system that induce vomiting.

Dying cells and the cells that eat them produce large amounts of certain proteins called interleukins that are normally involved in the body's defense against infections. Interleukins exert their effects by coupling with receptors on many cells and setting off a jangling of signals that can be lumped together under a general descriptive term called the inflammatory response. Though most of us are unaware of the intricate biochemistry of the inflammatory response, we all know it when we feel it during an infection. The fatigue, fever, weight loss, muscle aching, loss of appetite, and depression associated with infection are well known to all of us. Cancer patients undergoing chemotherapy directed against DNA are regularly visited with those symptoms.

After each dose of chemotherapy, millions of cells are killed. Hopefully a higher fraction of cancer cells than normal cells succumb. But they all release their interleukins, and the cells that sweep up the debris release them as well. Chemotherapy is equivalent to a very prolonged and moderately severe case of the flu. Some patients just want to go to bed and stay there until it's all over. Others soldier on. And there are long-term consequences. For example, chemotherapy and estrogen blockade may cause vaginal dryness, which inhibits sexuality.

Partridge had informed Joan about all of these symptoms, which Joan knew about anyway from her friends. She gritted her teeth and came for the first treatment. An attempt was made to start the first intravenous treatment, but her vein broke as the fluid began to run in. Fortunately, the Adriamycin, which is very toxic to tissues, had not yet been started. Partridge decided to give Joan a portacath, the same equipment used to treat Mario. Another accident ensued. The first port clotted and had to be replaced. Joan was not happy. She thought the surgeons who placed the port were not attentive to their work, as they were discussing football scores.

The story of the chatty surgeons irritated me when I heard about it. I don't know how many times hospitals warn staff members to remain professional in the presence of patients. One World War II axiom carries over to the war on cancer: loose lips sink ships. Stupid personal remarks in elevators and discussions of irrelevant entertainment in operating rooms, radiology suites, or around nursing stations destroy the morale of patients and families who expect physicians and nurses to be attentive to them and to the task at hand. Errors may be made. They are inevitable when thousands of procedures are performed. We cannot legislate against a technical failure. But we can maintain the morale of patients and family members by making sure that our actions persuade them that their needs are our sole concern. Malpractice suits are spawned when there is a combination of technical failure and apparent lack of interest. Joan is strong enough to deal with such episodes and forget about them. But another patient—one more frightened, more alone, and angrier— might have retaliated. I didn't report those surgeons to their chief. Perhaps I made a mistake.

The port finally placed, Joan received her first dose of Adriamycin and Cytoxan. She was successfully treated with intravenous and oral antiemetics and had very little trouble with vomiting during or immediately after her chemotherapy cycle. She was given copious amounts of fluids to dilute the Cytoxan in her urine so that it would not unduly injure her bladder cells. After having spent ten hours at Dana-Farber, Joan and her daughter, Ellen, who had accompanied her, finally went home.

The next morning, Joan awakened utterly drained of energy. She had prepared for the exhaustion and had a collection of Gregorian chants, classical symphonies, and inspirational tapes. She listened to them throughout the day for the next three months.

"I guess I decided to be in a space where I would do what I had to do and respond to how I was feeling but not get upset about it," Joan explained.

She didn't have to worry about Bob. Neighbors and friends took responsibility for him, bringing home-cooked meals that Joan picked at and Bob could guiltily enjoy.

"I would eat. I had a pretty good appetite. I tried to stay as cheerful as I could and have dinner with Bob and think about my wonderful friends and family. I refused to contemplate death. I know that cancer can lead to death, and I don't brush that aside. I know the reality of that, but I was never angry and I was never fearful. I guess it's because I realize death is inevitable and that it can happen to any of us at any time. But I know that there are people who think that cancer is a death sentence, and I don't see it that way anymore. Maybe I did when I first heard about it, but I realized how many people survive, and I wanted to work on being one of those survivors.

"I remember something you once told me—'We will take a year of your life for the rest of your life.' That was sage wisdom and set a tone for me in moving forward. But I was blessed with people around me who gave me good support."

With Ellen, Jeff, and Bob and her friends behind her, Joan kept those regular chemo appointments. She needed at least two and a half weeks to recover her strength after a course of treatment. By that time, she had to get organized for a return to Boston for the next dose. Aside from the total exhaustion and mild nausea, she lived through it. But there was one very frightening complication and plenty of minor ones.

The antivomiting medications are wonderful drugs, but all of them tend to cause constipation, and, as is true for many women, Joan has had trouble with constipation since going through childbirth. As Joan's white cell count fell, the germs in her large bowel multiplied and the bowel became inflamed. In the middle of the night, a few days following her first course of treatment, Joan awakened with severe pain in her belly. She had a slight fever as well. Fortunately, Partridge had kept Joan's local physician well informed. Bob rushed her to the local hospital, where she was held in the emergency department and sent to Brigham and Women's Hospital the next day with a diagnosis of acute colitis. Treatment with antibiotics and stool softeners fixed the problem, and she had no further crises. But she remembers the panic and the awful uncertainty of that night.

Perhaps it was that episode more than any that bonded her tightly to Partridge. The only truly happy events surrounding her regular visits to the "Borgia Palace," as Joan nicknamed Dana-Farber, were her visits with Partridge. During those visits, Partridge successfully encouraged her to take Taxol with her radiation therapy and therefore to come to Boston for the combined treatment.

"You have a pretty aggressive cancer. We need to put everything we can toward getting rid of it."

Joan agreed and made up her mind to continue to do everything she could to beat the odds. She completed her Adriamycin/Cytoxan in December, took a two-week holiday, and then wonderful friends invited her to live with them in their apartment in Boston so that she could have her daily radiation therapy punctuated by Taxol infusions. Her hair fell out, but she didn't bother with a wig. She wore hats and kerchiefs and looked forward to its return. She would have radiation therapy five days a week for six weeks during which she would have two treatments with Taxol and then two more doses of Taxol separated by three weeks. She could return to her home for the weekends. All this would take place from January through March. Then she would be through with all of the treatment except for the hysterectomy and ovary removal that would follow a few months later and five years of tamoxifen.

Before Joan began her six-week course of radiation therapy, I talked to Jay Harris, the chief of radiation oncology and the physician described by Iglehart as "the man who wrote the book on breast cancer." Harris emphasized that the role of radiation therapy is to achieve local control of breast cancer while chemotherapy and hormone receptor blockade with tamoxifen contribute to local and distant control. Radiation therapy focuses on the chest wall and the armpit, avoiding the sites in the armpit that were dissected by the surgeon. The avoidance is necessary to prevent a common unpleasant complication: arm edema (swelling due to obstruction of lymph channels). So the radiation oncologist and the surgeon must have a very close collaborative arrangement—one that Harris readily achieves with Iglehart.

The heart must also be excluded from the radiation beams in order to prevent early onset of coronary artery damage. The decision to apply radiation therapy in lymph node–positive breast cancer is still somewhat controversial even though several clinical trials have supported its use. Harris is cautious about its value and very mindful of its risks, but he is convinced that women like Joan, with large primary tumors and four or more positive lymph nodes in the armpit, undoubtedly have a lower recurrence incidence in the margins of the surgical field (called local control) and very likely have a better overall survival if they receive radiation.

The exact application of the beam is the intellectual and technical challenge of radiation oncology. Patients are placed in a mold that holds them in a precise and completely reproducible position. With the aid of a computer, the radiation machine, called a linear accelerator, delivers high-energy waves of varying tissue penetrance to a precisely mapped target. The planning of the energies and their distribution to the target is first accomplished in a simulation of the treatment using CT scans. In Joan's case, four different fields of treatment were to be delivered in each session. The multiple doses spread over a long period were chosen to avoid excessive radiation toxicity. The development of this complex therapeutic plan was the result of collaboration among radiation physicists, oncologists, imaging scientists, and skilled technicians.

Harris, who is a major international leader in breast cancer treatment, is particularly excited about new approaches to radiation therapy using high-speed computers and special focusing devices that will allow the therapist to literally paint a particular area of the body with radiation. The technique is called intensity modulated radiation or IMR. It will soon supplant the "old" methods that Joan received and reduce radiation toxicity even further. This will allow more of the energy to be delivered to suspected areas of residual disease, such as the margins of the surgery, without damaging normal tissues. He also looks forward to the use of cancer genetics rather than counting lymph nodes in the armpit as the most appropriate guide to therapy. If the work of Stephen Friend and his colleagues at Rosetta ImPharmatics and in the Netherlands can be extended—work that was the first to demonstrate that the pattern of gene expression in breast cancer predicts metastasis—Harris will make future decisions that will be far less arbitrary than a lymph node count.

Jay Harris and his team of physicians, nurses, and radiation therapists joined Partridge to care for Joan in January. She had moved into her friends' apartment in Boston and was ready for the next phase of her treatment. Joan became a daily visitor to Dana-Farber and plunged into the complementary therapy program. She felt well enough to participate because she tolerated the radiation treatments extremely well with very little irritation of the skin. In fact, she actually enjoyed the radiation therapy community, explaining, "That's a special little corner down there, and it is filled with patients, excellent technicians, and supportive nurses. The patients get to know one another and chat with each other because we are all there at a regular time. And there is always some kind of food or a puzzle or something to keep us all busy."

Joan was so invested in complementary therapy that she urged her radiation oncology nurse to let her teach the relaxation response to patients who became anxious in the radiation oncology waiting room. In effect, Joan combined the enterprises, having radiation treatment in the morning and Reiki massages, nutrition seminars, relaxation tapes, and labyrinth walks in the afternoon. Fearful of a recurrence of her colitis, she paid careful attention to her own nutrition, particularly the types of fat and fiber in her diet, and she was fascinated by claims that fish oil, soy, ginger, green tea, and pomegranates may reduce the risk of cancer. She listened to tapes by Belleruth Naparstek and Bernard Siegel and read books by Rabbi Abraham Jacobs Heschel and Rachel Naomi Remen. In effect, she never lost control of her care or her dignity as an individual. She marched through Taxol and radiation therapy with a minimum of toxicity except that the Taxol did catch up with her peripheral nerves. She had burning discomfort on the soles of her feet and trouble with her gait for months after the Taxol treatment. "I felt I was walking on bubble wrap."

But Joan surmounted the Taxol as well. That next summer, six months after she had completed her treatment, she was out on her beloved golf course. She was taking tamoxifen, the estrogen receptor blocker that she would take for the next five years. She couldn't walk the course because of the Taxol-induced neuropathy; she needed a cart, but she was out there with her lovely smile and cheery greeting, her hair obviously beginning to regrow. I saw her early in the summer and asked her how she was doing. I mentioned that she has wonderful friends and family who love her very much and helped to bring her through. Joan agreed that her friends and family made it all possible, but she wanted me to know that she was grateful to the Dana-Farber staff members, who had done their best to help her, and her eyes misted when she mentioned Partridge, to whom she had bonded so tightly. I decided to talk to Partridge about that relationship.

Ann Partridge was obviously close to Joan. The two women had connected at their first meeting even though theirs was a professional relationship. Partridge's first task was to be sure that Joan understood and accepted all of the therapy that was piled on her. The Taxol decision was a hard one but important, because a large clinical trial had demonstrated a small but definite advantage of Taxol in women with lymph node–positive stage 3A breast cancer. Partridge realized that Joan's trust in her had allowed Joan to get over her fear of the drug in order to have the best chance for success. She felt sorry that Joan had several relatively minor difficulties, among them an irregular heartbeat that was stress related, an increased incidence of migraine headaches, and mild arm swelling, which she treated with massage and exercise. She also noted knee pain and swelling due to a torn meniscus and wondered whether Taxol played a role. But, obviously, there are too many torn menisci in non-Taxol-treated patients to blame the drug for that complaint.

Partridge spoke thoughtfully about Joan. "I think she saw me as her caregiver, helping to manage her care in terms of the smaller things. We bonded from the beginning. She's a lovely person and she was easy to care for. She had a lot of little things that came up, and she continues to have mean little things that come up. She needs a fair bit of reassurance, and I can provide that most of the time. As you know, when people go on to survive breast cancer, there is always a risk of recurrence, and that can be terrifying. The first bit of arthritis a woman gets following a diagnosis of breast cancer is very likely to convince her that she has a bone metastasis. Joan's had a few episodes of things like that since her active treatment has been completed, but we have navigated through them."

I asked Partridge whether she ever worries about getting breast cancer herself. And I wondered how she handled emotional attachment to patients whom she might lose. "Yes, I worry about getting breast cancer, and I do all the appropriate things I recommend to patients about screening for breast cancer and thinking about breast cancer. But I don't obsess about it. I don't worry too much because I think I'd drive myself crazy. And I know how much I relate to my patients and how bad I feel if I lose one. I particularly worry about that with Joan, because I have developed such a bond with her. I saw her very frequently initially; she's invited me to go to her summer home. I hug her when I see her. I have several patients like her to whom I feel very close, and so the protective part of me says, 'Don't get too close to this person.' But that's not my personality really. I can't do that. And so I end up getting close to people. Hopefully, Joan will do fine, and if she doesn't, then I'll see her through that."

At the time of this conversation, Partridge had not lost any patients who began with stage 3 disease or less. But she was realistic. She knew that she would lose one-fifth of them in time. That, of course, is very much better than my initial experience in which over half of my stage 3 breast cancer patients were lost, usually quite quickly. None of my patients with leukemia survived. It is harder for physicians like Partridge to lose a patient because the losses are quite rare and the bonds correspondingly deeper.

Partridge's father and sister are very active general surgeons. She has great admiration for her father and surely was influenced by him to become a physician. Married and the mother of three small children, she must find a way to balance her home and professional life. I really do not know how these young women do it. Sometimes I think they do it with mirrors. I deeply admire them.

I asked Partridge to tell me what she would offer Joan if she did relapse. I wanted to know what was in her bag of tricks. I had had a recent conversation about the nature of relapse in breast cancer with Eric Winer and Jonathan Fletcher, a very experienced pathologist. The two warned me that relapse in breast cancer usually represents the resurgence of the same clone of breast cancer cells that started the disease but with enough genetic modifications to persuade both of them that the resurgent tumor is often a subset of the original clone. The chromosomes may differ, and a formerly estrogen receptor–positive tumor may occasionally reappear as negative. And even if it remains estrogen receptor positive, it may no longer require estrogen for growth. Hence it is unresponsive to tamoxifen or the newer aromatase inhibitors.

My discussion with Partridge took place after the results of two recently conducted clinical trials had been released. On the strength of those trials, Joan would not stop therapy after five years of tamoxifen. She would be placed on an aromatase inhibitor for a protracted period after tamoxifen had been completed. Aromatase is the enzyme in body fat, the liver, and the adrenal glands that converts androgen to estrogen.

Partridge reminded me that relapse in breast cancer does not have the connotation of imminent doom that is the case of relapse in lung and some other cancers. There are plenty of options, and it is possible to live reasonably comfortably for years with the disease. If, for example, Joan's disease recurred on or after the aromatase inhibitor, Partridge might add fulvestrant (Faslodex), another ER inhibitor.

The most exciting new option is certainly Herceptin (trastuzumab) for Her2/neu-positive patients. But that monoclonal antibody inhibitor of a receptor tyrosine kinase is only effective in the 20 percent of patients who express the enzyme. Recently, the pharmaceutical company GlaxoSmithKline released a small molecule called lapatinib that blocks the Her2/neu type of growth factor. That drug is now being tested in clinical trials. Whether it will be generally as effective as the antibody Herceptin is not presently known, but it may have the additional advantage of penetration into the brain, and many Her2/neu-positive patients suffer from brain metastases. Joan is one of the 80 percent who are Her2/neu negative, and breast cancers do not change their Her2/neu status when and if they relapse, but lapatinib represents further evidence of progress in smart drug development.

Vinorelbine (Navelbine) is another relatively new chemotherapeutic drug. It works in cells like Taxol, but it is less neurotoxic than Taxol. It has been used with Herceptin in most settings but could be used with other drugs as well.

Capecitabine (Xeloda), an oral chemotherapeutic drug, is another option. In the body, capecitabine converts to 5-fluorouracil, an old standby that inhibits the folic acid pathway. But the drug seems to be quite active against metastatic disease, and it is reasonably well tolerated.

Several new folic acid pathway inhibitors are now in trials and appear encouraging. They are not smart drugs because they affect a pathway that is required by cancer and normal cells alike, but they are effective in some cases.

Partridge emphasized again that you have to be persistent in the treatment of relapsed breast cancer and move from one treatment to another, sometimes over a very long time. "I just had a woman see me who's now ten years out from her initial diagnosis of metastatic disease. She's been on several clinical trials and obviously she's still alive and been doing okay. She's someone who always says, 'Bring on the trial,' because she's had good responses to things in the past and she's always willing to try something that may be the thing that keeps her disease in check for a longer period of time."

Partridge is completely correct. Relapsed breast cancer is usually a chronic illness. Occasionally it runs wild in patients for reasons we do not understand. Winer calls that rare event "leukemia of the breast." When it happens, it's dreadful, but it is very rare. Most of the time, breast cancer is simply a chronic war, and the question is how do you get patients to fight that war without beating them up in the process, without forcing them to be chronic losers in the campaign?

I ask my patients with cancer to act like football tackles. Those tackles are very large people who simply walk forward. They never look to the left or the right. That's not their job description. They take one or two yards at a time until they hit the goal line. I think the much smaller women with breast cancer have to emulate their bulky football brethren. They have to have that mind-set. They can't look around too much. If they do look around, they begin to get very nervous. But if they keep their head down and just march forward, they can get through the weeks, the months, and the years. And it is often many, many years.

So we cannot let our patients get panicky. If they do, they may be panicky for decades. I've known patients with metastatic breast cancer for fifteen years. They may reach their life expectancy with breast cancer. If we cannot cure them, we must try to give them a decent and productive life expectancy. Right now that is seventy-seven years. It seems to me that if doctors can get their relapsed patients functioning well and living to age seventy-seven, much of the battle has been won, even if the disease is still present. And if the patient is fortunate enough to have a physician like Ann Partridge, the battle is half won before it starts.

Finally, many patients with breast cancer find a new meaning in life after they have gone through the purgatory of therapy. As Joan once told me, "I am blessed with wonderful friends and family. I am so grateful for the love that came to me. My friend, Janet, calls cancer a gift. I'm not ready to call it a gift, but I am ready to say that it brings good things to you. It has changed my life for the better. I haven't enjoyed my aches and pains, but I think I have learned to love more because of this. And I do feel that love surrounded me. I don't want to be too sentimental, but that's the way I handled it."

# CHAPTER FIFTEEN

# The Future of Epithelial Cancer Therapy

The goal of cancer research is to improve our ability to prevent and cure epithelial cancers like breast cancer. Though our achievements in cancer prevention are less than impressive, Mario's and Joan's stories show that we have made great progress in curing patients. But even in childhood leukemia and stage 3A breast cancer, two types of cancer that are very responsive to modern treatment, we only cure 80 percent of those who are afflicted. That is a huge increase in the cure rate over the nearly fifty years of my experience, but it isn't good enough. We need much more understanding of epithelial cancer biology if we are to develop the treatments that will capture the last 20 percent.

Fortunately, we are gaining that vital knowledge. Cancer is an acquired genetic disease, and we are learning a vast amount about the human genome. As a result, we know much more about the genetic changes that cause cancer. From that knowledge we will gain new and much smarter therapeutic options and have them ready should Mario or Joan relapse. In fact, we already have a very new and effective smart drug in reserve for Mario should he need it. What about Joan? Keeping in mind that her cancer is Her2/neu negative and therefore ineligible for Herceptin or lapatinib—the leading smart treatment for breast cancer today—can we hope for something new that would help her if she relapses somewhere down the line?

Though we lack another general-purpose smart drug for breast cancer at this moment, we are gathering information that will lead to better drugs in the near future. We are learning much more about the precise genetic events that turn a normal cell into a cancer cell. Much of that information has come from Robert Weinberg's laboratory at MIT. Weinberg and Bill Hahn, now at Dana-Farber, have shown that a normal epithelial cell can be turned into a malignant tumor if certain genes are altered. Among the several requirements are high expression of genes like ras that hasten the rate of cell division, another gene called telomerase that prevents the usual erosion of tips of chromosomes during cell division, and defective expression of the genes that produce the sniffing proteins that detect and send damaged cells down the death pathway. Cancer is the result of too much division *and* too little death.

Weinberg and Hahn's work suggests that several defective genes operate in a coordinated way to cause cancer. That is a worry. It will be very hard to define drugs that will interfere with several different pathways, all of which are responsible for parts of the problem. But both Bob Weinberg and Francis Collins, the latter the director of the National Human Genome Research Institute of the National Institutes of Health, are optimistic that the extensive mutation injury to cancer cell DNA actually creates Achilles' heels in the cells. The mutations increase several drivers of cell division and eliminate important death pathways. In so doing, they turn cancer cells into growing machines, but the cancer cells become absolutely dependent on one or two of those changes in pathways. They cannot survive without them. If we can define and block those acquired pathways, we can hoist the cancer cells on their own petards.

Francis Collins is a tall, well-spoken North Carolinian. He was a chemistry major at the University of North Carolina who got a Ph.D. in quantum mechanics—about as far from cancer as you can get in science. In the middle of his Ph.D. training, he discovered molecular biology and genetics and decided to change his career. The genetics program at Yale is particularly strong, so he made his way to New Haven for research training in a laboratory directed by one of my former Harvard Medical School classmates who told me that Collins was one of the best he had ever seen. I met him and totally agreed. I've admired Collins since he began his medical research career. I've particularly admired his determination to give something back to society. Every summer, until the past few, Collins has volunteered as a physician in a clinic in an underdeveloped country. He doesn't talk about that commitment. He just does it.

After Yale, Collins went on to the University of Michigan, where he led the team that discovered the gene defect in cystic fibrosis, a severe inherited pulmonary and gastrointestinal tract disease of children and young adults. Several years ago, Collins was asked to head the human genome project at the National Institutes of Health. That enormous international task, the base-by-base sequencing of the entire human genome, was substantially completed in 2000, well ahead of schedule and actually underbudget. Now Collins is the director of the National Human Genome Research Institute at the National Institutes of Health.

Despite his numerous responsibilities, Collins continues to operate a research laboratory and has found a beautiful example of the Achilles' heel of epithelial cancer. There is a rare human epithelial cancer called multiple endocrine neoplasia. Patients with this type of cancer get malignant tumors in the insulin-producing islets of the pancreas, in the pituitary, and in other endocrine glands. The tumors have multiple genetic abnormalities and have the highly damaged chromosomes that characterize breast cancer and other epithelial cancers even in their earliest stages. One of those gene defects stands out. It is a missing or defective gene that Collins calls MEN1. Collins has developed a mouse model of the human disease. When he reinserts that gene in its normal form into tumors, they disappear. So MEN1 is an antioncogene such as the breast cancer–associated (BRCA) genes or p53.

Though the genome of multiple endocrine neoplasia tumors is badly damaged and bears many defects, restoration of only one defective gene cures the tumor. From this important observation and several others like it, we have to conclude that a search of tumors for their Achilles' heels, or what we might also call the soft underbelly of cancer, must reveal the pathways that smart drugs can successfully attack.

With quiet determination, Nellie Polyak, the young investigator at Dana-Farber who demonstrated that *normal* breast cells may become chemically modified and support the growth of cancer cells, is pursuing the soft underbelly of breast cancer cells themselves. Polyak was born in Hungary and knew she wanted to be a scientist from the moment she gave up her dolls. Her grandparents were German Jews who barely escaped the Nazis, fled to Hungary, and survived the savagery of World War II. Her grandmother actually immigrated to the United States to become a nurse at a hospital in Boston.

Polyak went on to the university in Szeged as a medical student, where professors noticed her penchant for and nascent skill in research. She was sent as a special student to do laboratory research at the Hungarian National Academy of Sciences, where she became committed to a career in cancer research. Knowing that Hungary had a severely underfunded research base, she elected to seek graduate training in the United States. After she received her medical degree in Hungary, Polyak attended the graduate school of medical sciences at Cornell and the Sloan Kettering Institute in New York City. She had made a commitment to basic laboratory research.

Polyak had a spectacular career in New York and received a coveted postgraduate training opportunity in Bert Vogelstein's laboratory at Johns Hopkins University. Vogelstein, a physician scientist, had pioneered a highly successful inquiry into the genetic basis of colon cancer. He is one of the fathers of cancer genetics. Vogelstein insists that his graduate and postdoctoral students visit the cancer clinics so that they can understand the importance of their work.

The patients made an indelible impression on Polyak. She competed successfully for a junior faculty position at Dana-Farber and began her work on the genetic basis of breast cancer. Polyak knew that she would contribute in the laboratory and not in the clinic, but she wanted to see the patients coming through the front door of the cancer center. Like her mentor, Vogelstein, she knew that the sight of them would encourage her trainees to work as hard as possible to find biological principles about breast cancer that could be rapidly translated into new therapies.

Polyak's first approach was to collect as many samples as possible of the different presentations of breast cancer—from ductal carcinoma in situ (DCIS), the preinvasive lesion that arises from one mutated duct lining or epithelial cell and remains entirely in the ductal system, to broadly invasive disease. To gather the samples, she needed the cooperation of several breast surgeons like Dirk Iglehart and the all-important pathologists who understand the anatomic as well as the genetic details of breast cancer.

Having collected the samples, Polyak asked a simple question: What are the genes that are uniquely expressed in DCIS, and are they different in invasive breast cancer? To answer the question, Polyak adopted a method of analysis of gene expression that differs from the microarray technique that Todd Golub utilized when he and Scott Armstrong found the aberrant flt3 overexpression in Mario's MLL leukemia. Microarray analysis tests the *relative* expression of certain previously identified genes in two or more tissues or cancers. The method that Polyak adopted is called serial analysis of gene expression (SAGE). It identifies the *absolute* amount of expression of genes within a given tissue or a nodule of cancer.

Within a two-year period, Polyak found two very important gene expression abnormalities in breast cancer. The first discovery was a gene called hin1. (Hin is an acronym for "high in normal.") The hin gene produces a growth-regulating protein that is very readily detectable in normal duct cells and almost entirely lost in DCIS or invasive breast cancer. It seems to act like another antioncogene.

The second discovery is even more exciting. Polyak found overexpression of a gene called ibc1 (the acronym for "invasive breast cancer") in the ductal cells of patients with highly invasive large breast cancers that metastasize early. The gene was not previously identified in the human genome. It produces a growth-promoting protein that acts like a dominant oncogene. Obviously we need much more information about it and its receptor because it might be possible to develop an assay for its function, and from that technology, create a drug that would inhibit the growth-promoting function of the protein and stop invasive breast cancer in its tracks.

Polyak knows the importance of her work. She is in the lab night and day trying to get the data on ibc1 as rapidly as possible because she sees Joan and the hundreds of other women coming through the doors of the cancer center every day. The physician in her wants to help them. She takes time off to create some lovely impressionist paintings of neighboring brooks and footbridges. That releases her tensions and clears her mind. Then she can return to the work with fresh resolve.

Polyak and other committed scientists worldwide are determined to find the pathways of breast cancer cells and shut them down with smart drugs. Joan, the thousands of patients like her, and their families are relying on the discovery of such drugs.

Meanwhile, Joan is back at work on community development projects. We all hope that her breast cancer treatment is now behind her, but we continue to search for the smart drugs that will totally eradicate her disease and the breast cancer that plagues thousands of women every year. Given sufficient time and effort, we will find them.

# Ken's Story

# CHAPTER SIXTEEN

# The Explosion

Ken was built like a fireplug. His neck was short and solidly planted on broad shoulders. He had a barrel chest that formed a fairly neat rectangle with his prominent abdomen, which stood over two short, powerful legs. I had a few inches on Ken, but his compact build and the firm grip of his hand left the sound impression that I would fare poorly in a physical contest against him. Ken, who moved quickly and gracefully and whose bright eyes darted around to take in new surroundings, had been wrestling for years. I wrestled as a high school student, but this fellow would have made mincemeat out of me in a few seconds.

I met Ken because he had a type of cancer that was absolutely untreatable until just a few years ago. He had a highly aggressive sarcoma, a type of cancer that can afflict muscles, nerves, and bone, as well as fat, cartilage, and fibrous tissue. In Ken's case, the previously untreatable cancer involved his gastrointestinal tract and is known as GIST, which stands for gastrointestinal stromal tumor.

Though GIST is a relatively uncommon tumor, its behavior and the challenges posed by its treatment provide an excellent model for figuring out new treatments for the common cancers such as breast, prostate, lung, and colon. A cancer treatment revolution and a great attitude were critical as Ken dealt with GIST—and the same tools and attitudes will be critical for managing more common cancers, particularly when they are resistant to classic chemotherapy treatments.

Ken, who was born in the Bronx in 1949, had cancer in his family history, but nothing that would suggest he would end up with GIST. His mother died from lung cancer, and her mother had liver cancer, but undoubtedly those cases resulted from environmental factors: heavy smoking and alcoholism. Ken's love of wrestling in high school and his coaching that sport later on helped him avoid those habits, but nothing could prevent a single cell in his gastrointestinal tract from undergoing a mutation that led to his cancer.

Although he was overweight, Ken never had health problems until GIST began to manifest itself. He regularly walked five miles, had normal blood pressure and cholesterol, and felt well. His marriage with Peggy, who had been his sweetheart since they were eleven years old, was ideal. They had a son and a daughter and were grandparents. Ken, a salesman, said his work was wonderful and that his fellow employees at a Massachusetts manufacturing company were great to him. With two secure incomes, a nearly paid-for home, and good health insurance, Ken and Peggy were very happy.

In 1998, Ken began to notice some weakness and mild shortness of breath when he walked briskly or climbed a flight of stairs. The symptoms were slowly but inexorably progressing. Ken reported them to his primary physician, who tested his blood and found him to be anemic, meaning that his red blood cell and circulating hemoglobin counts were low. While the normal level of hemoglobin for a man of his age ranges from 12 to 16 grams for every 3 ounces of blood, Ken's hemoglobin count was only 6 grams. He was very anemic, and he was becoming tired quite easily.

His primary physician referred him to a blood specialist, who noted that Ken's red blood cells looked as though he had become iron deficient. The blood specialist decided to treat him with iron. But the doctor told Ken that his case was puzzling. Iron deficiency does not occur out of the blue. If adults have normal levels of iron at one point in time and are deficient at another, they must have bled at some point to account for the lower iron level, since bleeding is the only way to eliminate iron from the body.

The only site for significant but invisible bleeding in men is the gastrointestinal tract. If a doctor sees a man with iron deficiency of unknown cause, then he or she must hunt for blood in the stool. Blood would have leaked from somewhere in the twenty-five feet of intestines. Next, the physician must use all available methods to explore the gastrointestinal tract and locate the bleeding point.

Ken's specialist repeatedly tested Ken's stools for blood, but he could not find any trace of it. Then he made a mistake. Instead of concluding that his diagnosis must be flawed, he decided to treat Ken with iron, believing that the blood loss must be subtle and that his tests had simply missed it. The treatment, he thought, would replace the iron Ken had supposedly lost by bleeding.

Most of good medical care is built on a solid basis of paranoia. Doctors must always suspect that someone or something is out to get their patients. The best physicians always live suspiciously, questioning their diagnoses and whether their patients are following necessary instructions. Outstanding doctors continuously ask questions. The art of medicine lies in invisible suspicion and silent self-criticism.

Ken turned out to fall into the group of one of every ten patients who seems to have iron deficiency yet is not bleeding. When people have chronic inflammation from an abscess, rheumatoid arthritis, colitis, or large tumor, the body withholds iron from the blood. In those conditions, the liver overproduces a small signaling protein, which then acts as an instructor. It commands the storage cells in the body that normally release iron into the blood to hold tightly to the metal. The lack of iron in the blood starves the newly formed blood cells; in turn, the patients become anemic. Ken had no obvious abscess on his body, was free of rheumatoid arthritis and colitis, and showed no external signs of having a tumor. So the hematologist did not worry sufficiently about those possibilities.

If the hematologist had been more critical of his own reasoning and used modern imaging techniques such as computerized tomography (CT) to make a clear picture of the organs in his patient's abdomen, he might have correctly diagnosed the situation and prevented what would become a disaster. Unbeknownst to Ken or his doctors, a mass of rapidly dividing cancer cells was emerging from his small intestine in the form of a growing tumor. The cancer cells were releasing proteins that circulate and interrupt many normal body systems. One or more of those proteins entered the liver and instructed it to release a large amount of the signaling protein that blocks iron from returning to the blood from storage cells. Therefore, Ken developed all the signs of iron deficiency anemia even though he had plenty of iron in his body. The iron was locked up in his storage cells.

When iron pills did not correct Ken's anemia and he became weaker, he started receiving repeated red blood cell transfusions. That decision alarmed Ken's primary physician, who insisted on further inquiry. Ken had a colonoscopy, but it too was unrevealing. Unfortunately, the primary physician was not quite suspicious enough. Like the specialist, he did not order a CT scan of Ken's abdomen.

Two years later, Ken talked to me about his reaction to the mistaken diagnosis. "I think we have a responsibility to ourselves in every way, but [in the past] I forfeited that when it came to medical matters. In every other area of my life—financially, intellectually, spiritually, and emotionally—I always took care of myself and took responsibility for myself. When it came to the possibility of the physical end of my life, I abdicated. I simply said, 'These people have degrees; I'm going to trust them.'"

For nearly a year, Ken continued the blood transfusion and iron regimen without incident. He followed his regular routine, rising early for a brisk walk, coming back to the house for breakfast, hugging his wife, and setting off to do his rounds as an expert salesman. In July 1999, Peggy went on vacation with a few friends, the first vacation she had taken without Ken in six years. Two nights later, disaster struck.

In the middle of the night, Ken was awakened because he felt a "pop" in his abdomen. Suddenly he had terrible abdominal pain. His stomach muscles contracted violently and became rigid. He tried to roll into a ball to relieve the pain, but it began to consume him. He shrieked in pain and terror and broke out into an enormous sweat that soaked the sheets in seconds. Then he started to lose consciousness as his blood pressure began to collapse. Ken was going into shock, but he had the presence of mind to grab the phone from the bedside table and call 911. The details are hazy after that.

He groaned his name and address to the operator and told her he thought he was dying. The operator told him to stay on the phone and talk to her until the ambulance could get to him. She kept talking and making him answer. Ken lay on his side, the phone under his left ear. He was listening to the operator and trying to respond as he pressed his knees into his chest to stop the terrible pain. The operator promised him relief in a few moments. Then the pain seemed to recede and he became drowsy, his lips and tongue thick, with a cottony feeling in his mouth. Ken began to mutter incoherently. He couldn't get words out. He whispered into the phone.

He began hearing waves on a shore and then high-pitched shrieking that turned into a loud wail and interrupted the gentle sound of the waves. Outside, an ambulance and police escort car had arrived. EMTs piled out and pounded on the door, but Ken, slipping into a coma, could hear only a faint tapping. A big cop jumped out of the cruiser, ran to the front door, and lifted his foot with its thick-soled boot. One kick and he broke the door open.

The EMTs dashed into the house and ran up the stairs to the bedroom, where they found Ken babbling incoherently. They saw him rolled up in the soaked sheets, sweat still pouring from his body. His bowels had opened and he was smeared with feces. They could feel a pulse at the neck, but his blood pressure was almost unobtainable. His belly was as hard as a board. They knew immediately that Ken was dying of an abdominal catastrophe.

They used the sheets to clean him off, rolled him over, and miraculously found a healthy vein in his forearm. They pushed in a needle and began a rapid infusion of a water, glucose, and salt solution. Then they bundled Ken onto a stretcher, brought him out to the ambulance, and sped off to the local community hospital. On the way, they added a bottle of a normal plasma protein called albumin to the intravenous treatment. They hoped the substance would help to maintain Ken's blood volume and keep him out of irreversible shock.

A sudden abdominal catastrophe is often caused by a broken segment of intestine—for example, due to a ruptured appendix or gallbladder. Rapid inflammation of the pancreas or a torn blood vessel—for instance, the aorta (the body's major artery)—can also cause this emergency. But the EMTs were in no position to diagnose just what was happening. They needed to get Ken into a hospital where a surgeon could quickly open his abdomen, find the problem, and treat it.

Ken was lucky. The surgeon on call for emergencies was one of the best on the staff and would be considered excellent in any hospital, large or small. The disaster that befell Ken is a perfect illustration of the need for community hospitals that can deal with serious medical problems. His state of shock would have become irreversible in a few more minutes; he never would have stayed alive long enough for the ambulance to reach an urban teaching hospital.

Part of the huge cost of American medicine is its reliance on local community hospitals to deliver much more than standard routine care. Having a staff and maintaining the equipment needed for dealing with a crisis like Ken's may not be necessary more than two or three times a year. One of the central issues that affects the debate on health care costs in the United States is that this system is tremendously inefficient, yet it seems justified if the life saved happens to be your own or that of someone you love.

The surgeon who took care of Ken that night had about two minutes to make a decision. One look convinced him that Ken was suffering from a severe inflammation of the abdominal cavity called peritonitis. The surgeon was convinced that the contents of the bowel were pouring into Ken's belly. The cavity's normally thin, glistening lining—called the peritoneum—was severely inflamed, and the abdomen was beginning to swell from fluid and gas. Ken needed immediate surgery to clean out the abdomen and close the hole in his bowel. Ken also urgently required blood, intravenous fluids, and massive doses of antibiotics to quell the infection and inflammation in his abdomen.

In that brief period, the surgeon had to consider whether the dangerous condition might be the result of an intestinal hole, such as from a ruptured appendix, which is typical, or an acute inflammation of the pancreas. The latter condition releases digestive enzymes into the abdominal cavity, often causing enormous pain and inflammation. But such inflammation usually starts at a low level and builds up. Ken had become desperately ill almost immediately, suggesting that a hole had suddenly opened up in his bowel. The surgeon knew that the diagnosis was critical, because pancreatitis should be treated without surgery, if at all possible.

Deciding that Ken was more likely having a bowel catastrophe, the surgeon prepared him for immediate anesthesia, blood transfusion, and surgery. No time was available to wait for the results of imaging assays like routine X-rays or CT scans. The doctor also couldn't wait for the results of blood tests to rule out pancreatitis. He had to rely on a physical examination, his experience, and his skills.

As soon as Ken's belly was opened, the surgeon realized that his overall diagnosis was correct. He was certain that a hole had opened in Ken's small bowel, because the belly cavity was filled with gas and greenish foul-smelling fluid that could only come from the contents of the bowel. The surgeon learned exactly what was happening when he sucked out buckets of the mess. The appendix was normal, but a grapefruit-size tumor was growing out of the small bowel. The cells in the center of the tumor had died, and the bowel wall under those cells had virtually lique-fied, leaving a large hole through which the bacterial-laden bowel con-tents were pouring into the abdomen. Along with bacteria, the cancer cells that had formed the tumor had been spreading throughout the belly.

After cleaning out the cavity, the surgeon began the delicate process of removing the tumor and the eighteen inches of small intestinal seg-ment to which it was attached. He sewed the severed ends of the small intestine together to maintain its continuity. He repeatedly washed and sucked out any remaining loose contents of the cavity, trying to remove some of the bacteria and cancer cells that had spread widely in the area. He counted on a high level of intravenous antibiotics to finish the job on the bacteria. But he feared that one or more—perhaps many more—of the loose cancer cells would find a niche somewhere in the abdomen and begin to replicate. Ken was at risk of developing multiple tumor nodules within his belly.

The surgeon had no idea about the type of cancer he had removed and no confidence that any drug available to him would kill the spilled residual cells. He had to hope that mechanical flushing of the cavity would remove the cells. But he knew from experience that rupture of an abdominal tumor nearly always leads to the growth of multiple tumors around the abdomen. After doing the best he could, and confident that Ken's blood pressure could be maintained, he sewed up the incision he had made and sent Ken to the recovery room.

Despite the excellence of that surgical care, Ken barely survived. One complication after another plagued his body. The inflammation of the peritoneum had roughened and scarred the smooth lining of the abdom-inal cavity, and the resulting scar tissue easily caught and obstructed loops of bowel. Blood vessels that fed the bowel also became obstructed, necessitating more surgery. That involved removing dead intestine and sewing a loop of the healthy part of the intestinal tract to Ken's stomach so that he could eat.

This fix worked reasonably well. Ken could eat food, but the surgery had made the wall of the small intestine stretch, which caused a reversal of the normal waves of contraction when Ken ate. After a meal, he would break into a sweat, suddenly feel nauseous, and start to vomit. It took several months for his digestive system to adjust to its reconstruction.

Dangerous complications also developed. Inflammation and multiple surgeries cause a large increase of many clotting proteins in the blood. Ken developed clots in his leg veins. Some broke off as embolisms and traveled into his lungs, obstructing blood flow, which could have led to sudden death by cardiac arrest. He required prolonged intravenous and oral drugs known as anticoagulants to block the action of the clotting proteins and clear his legs and lungs of the clots. And since such drugs induce a risk of gastrointestinal bleeding, he needed regular blood tests to ensure that the activity of his clotting system was reduced but not abolished. Weeks of anticoagulant drugs and related blood tests nearly destroyed the veins in his arms.

While Ken was fighting off the blood clots that had traveled to his lungs, his doctors and Peggy learned about the nature of his cancer. Having never seen anything quite like his kind of tumor, pathologists at his community hospital had sent slides made of slices of the mass to their counterparts at a larger hospital and to the Armed Forces Institute of Pathology in Washington, D.C. They thought the tumor looked like the kind that arises in supporting tissues such as muscle, tendon, and bone. These are called sarcomas. (The Greek words *sarkos* and *oma* mean "flesh" and "swelling," respectively, so these are tumors of the flesh or muscle.)

The system for diagnosing unusual surgical samples such as Ken's is quite good in the United States. Hospital pathologists can ask for help from colleagues, and if necessary, a national resource. The Armed Forces Institute of Pathology (AFIP) has a huge collection of samples and a list of experts who can identify almost anything. (In 2004, the federal government threatened to discontinue the Armed Forces Institute of Pathology's service to American physicians—a vastly shortsighted idea but consistent with the scientific myopia that has characterized the recent administration.)

Ken had an unusual sarcoma called a gastrointestinal stromal tumor (GIST). His surgeon and Peggy did not tell Ken about this while he was still very weak, because no effective treatment for GIST was known other than complete removal by surgery—and that opportunity had been lost when the tumor had ruptured. The doctors saw no reason to deliver bad news while Ken was trying to recover.

During that period, Ken began to gain weight again, having lost forty pounds. The apparent iron deficiency that had begun the nightmare had been corrected by removing the tumor. His body started to make red cells filled with hemoglobin. With good care from his doctors and Peggy's ceaseless monitoring, Ken slowly regained his strength and actually started to extend his short walks from around his room to trips down the hospital corridors.

After a few weeks, when the surgeon concluded that Ken was healthy enough to take the bad news, his doctors told him that he had an incurable cancer. Ken took it stoically. He was as tough a patient as he had been a wrestler.

But Peggy had been unwilling to accept that nothing more could be done. She had asked the blood specialist who originally missed the diagnosis for his opinion. He suggested that Ken should receive a combination of chemotherapy drugs, but that didn't satisfy her, for she had also searched the Internet for information about the disease. She read that no combination of standard anticancer drugs had been proven effective in treating GIST.

Having decided that she didn't want to deal with that specialist anymore, Peggy continued doing online research. She found an Internet article about the treatment of sarcomas by George Demetri at Dana-Farber. She called Demetri and made an appointment for her husband. Peggy was not going to give up without a fight.

# CHAPTER SEVENTEEN

# Cancerous Hens and Constipated Mice

When Ken was strong enough to contemplate a trip to Boston to see Demetri, he and Peggy were already more knowledgeable about gastrointestinal stromal tumors than most physicians are. And they wanted to learn much more. Ken rapidly became fascinated by the energy and expertise that Demetri and his team were pouring into sarcoma research.

For the moment, Ken did not need any treatment because he had no detectable disease. The cells that had been scattered around his abdomen when the tumor ruptured had not yet formed new cancers. But Ken knew that time would change the situation. Sooner or later, his abdomen would become full of GIST tumors, and they would kill him if they were not stopped in their tracks.

Demetri explained that the moment had come when the cause of GIST had been determined. Drugs that can kill the tumor were about to become available. Ken would soon be able to try a new drug that might combat GIST. The doctor's team was about to conduct tests on imatinib (Gleevec), which had just been tested successfully in chronic myelogenous leukemia (CML). Ken and Peggy became medical sponges, soaking up knowledge about GIST and Gleevec as fast as Demetri and the Internet could produce information.

The story about how GIST was identified, how Gleevec might ameliorate it, and the start of the present cancer treatment revolution has its roots in the nineteenth century when a strange cancer epidemic was repeatedly sweeping through U.S. poultry farms where hens were packed tightly together. Typically the affected birds would develop swollen bellies and gasp for breath. When the hens were cut open, their abdomens were full of masses of cells—cancers. Or, less commonly, the birds would grow large tumors on their wings. In most outbreaks the tumors seemed to be masses of white blood cells, but some of the time the tumors appeared to be sarcomas that grew out of the tendons and other supporting structures of the wings. Poultry farmers were desperate. When one bird developed a tumor, the whole flock would get cancer and die—an economic crisis for the producer.

The situation seemed insoluble, since no scientist had even considered that cancer could be infectious. Experts had only established that cancer is a disease that might be caused by an external toxin. "No relationship could be conceived to exist between the invisible viruses and the self-sufficient growth of cancer cells," George Klein of the Royal Karolinska Institute in Stockholm stated many decades later about the situation. (He said this to the distinguished assemblage before the presentation— made almost six decades later—of the 1966 Nobel Prize to Peyton Rous, who deciphered the case when the ravages were at full force.)

The mystery intrigued Rous, a doctor who had accepted a full-time appointment to direct cancer research at the newly created Rockefeller Institute of Medical Research in New York. (The institute would subsequently become Rockefeller University.) In 1910, Rous, who had been brought up with animals on a Texas cattle ranch, discovered that a virus apparently caused the cancer that afflicted the hens.

It is remarkable that Rous reached this conclusion, since the causes of cancer were virtually unknown at the time. The most relevant previous work was that of Theodor Boveri (1862–1915), a German biologist who had demonstrated that most cancer cells have abnormal chromosomes, the elements of heredity. Boveri's findings had suggested that cancer is due to mutations of genes.

Rous had started the work after a poultry farmer brought a cancerous chicken with a wing sarcoma to his new laboratory at Rockefeller. The researchers minced up the cancer and suspended the chopped cells in water. The mixture did not include any intact cells. Yet after Rous injected the material into the wings of normal chickens, they developed sarcomas, which meant the cells had to be associated with a tumor-causing agent.

Rous next fractionated the mixture of minced tumor cells by filtering it through progressively narrow filters. He kept filtering until the material did not show anything visible, even when viewed under a microscope. But chickens injected with the seemingly empty fluid also promptly developed tumors. Rous concluded that a virus—a particle so small it could pass through any filters to which he subjected the material—must be causing the tumors.

The report of Rous's experiment landed on the medical science community with a dull thud. No one doubted the result, but very few believed that a virus might cause cancer. And those who bought the argument figured that the virus must be restricted to birds. After all, Rous tried to do the same experiment with mouse and rat cancers, but he never saw the same result. Even fifteen years later, Alexis Carrel, a highly distinguished researcher at Rockefeller, dismissed Rous's results, ascribing them to the presence of some cancer-causing toxin such as arsenic in the extracts.

Finally, after many years and much more research, other scientists began to recognize that tumor viruses could cause some cancers in rats, mice, and even humans. At age eighty-seven, Peyton Rous was finally awarded a Nobel Prize for his discovery. (Ironically, Alan Hodgkin, Rous's son-in-law, shared a Nobel Prize three years earlier for his work in another field, nerve conduction.)

Though Rous's work was eventually vindicated, the mechanism by which the sarcoma virus (now known as the Rous sarcoma virus or RSV) actually causes cancer was unknown for many more years. An understanding of that mechanism was critical to investigators who hoped to find a way to kill off the cancer or sarcoma that might be related to it.

The effort to figure out the mechanism started in the late 1940s and early 1950s when Renatto Dulbecco and Salvador Luria, two Italian expatriates who later received Nobel Prizes, initiated basic research and training programs in molecular biology at Indiana University and later at the California Institute of Technology (Dulbecco) and the Massachusetts Institute of Technology (Luria). The scientists they trained, and in turn the students of those scientists, played key roles not only in the biology of RSV and the like but also in making major basic discoveries about proteins, genes, DNA, and the related structure RNA in the second half of the twentieth century. Because of that work, we know that our twenty thousand to twenty-five thousand genes (the exact number is still in question) are large molecules known as polymers. They are made of DNA and lie along stretches of chromosomes in the nucleus of cells. DNA produces very similar polymers known as RNA, which in turn engage the protein-making machinery in the cells. In that fashion, each gene produces an RNA copy, and the RNA produces the protein governed by the gene. A mutation in DNA thereby causes a mutation in its RNA and thus disturbance of the protein's structure—its sequence of building blocks called amino acids. The change in structure can alter the function of the protein and result in disease.

The importance of the molecular biology program at Indiana was at least twofold. Dulbecco and Luria focused on two types of tumor viruses: those made of DNA and those made of RNA. Furthermore, they and the scientists who at one time or another worked with them mentored several generations of researchers, some of whom eventually won Nobel Prizes. James Watson, who became famous for his work on determining the physical structure of DNA, for which he shared a Nobel Prize in 1962, began his training in that Indiana program.

In the mid-1960s, Howard Temin, trained by Dulbecco in California and, at the time, a faculty member at the University of Wisconsin, proposed a heretical notion. He argued that when an RNA tumor virus enters a host cell's nucleus, a viral enzyme transforms its RNA into DNA, which is then incorporated into the DNA of the host cell's chromosomes. The action forms new host genes, which in turn produce more viral RNAs and thus more viral particles that leave the cell and go on to infect other cells.

Temin's idea seemed preposterous: the central dogma of what became known as molecular biology had been that DNA makes RNA, which makes protein. Nobody of consequence thought RNA could produce DNA. But in the early 1970s, Temin and David Baltimore, who had also worked with Dulbecco in California before joining Luria's department at the Massachusetts Institute of Technology, separately and simultaneously discovered reverse transcriptase, the viral enzyme that converts RNA to DNA. The discovery exploded the dogma, explained the life cycle of RNA tumor viruses, earned Temin and Baltimore a Nobel Prize in 1975, and led Michael Bishop and Harold Varmus to solve the mechanism by which the Rous sarcoma virus causes cancer, for which they also received a Nobel Prize, in 1989.

Bishop and Varmus, two physician scientists at the University of California in San Francisco (UCSF), had had much of their scientific training at the National Institutes of Health (NIH) in Bethesda, Maryland. Varmus, the son of a Long Island physician and grandson of an immigrant hatter, and Bishop, the son of a Lutheran minister whose family lived for generations along the Susquehanna River in a small town near Gettysburg, Pennsylvania, met in California shortly after Bishop had established a laboratory at UCSF to study tumor viruses. Varmus, who had just completed his initial laboratory training at NIH, had gone on a backpacking trip to California, where he wanted to find a postdoctoral training fellowship. He met Bishop on that trip, and they decided to work together.

Using laborious methods that have been completely supplanted in the present era of molecular biology, Bishop and Varmus showed that at some time in the distant past a benign strain of the Rous virus had invaded and incorporated its three RNA genes into the DNA of the cells of a host chicken. To do so, the virus had to copy its RNA into DNA with the reverse transcriptase enzyme and insert that DNA into the chicken cell chromosomes.

Errors can happen when reverse transcriptase does its work because many steps are involved. What can go wrong will go wrong. At least once, the reverse transcriptase "forgot" its role and began to copy an RNA derived from a gene that belonged to the chicken. It then copied the chicken RNA incorrectly and inserted that incorrect copy into the host chicken cell's DNA. That left the cell with a DNA blueprint to fabricate a virus with four genes instead of three. The fourth abnormal gene produced a mutated protein that causes cells to proliferate wildly, resulting in cancer. Bishop and Varmus called the new cancer-causing gene src (pronounced sarc), because it was found in the mutant Rous sarcoma virus.

Src represented a new class of genes. Bishop and Varmus coined the term *oncogene* (meaning a tumor-causing gene) to describe the mutant src gene and others in that class. And they firmly established that the src oncogene arises from a perfectly normal cellular src gene they called a proto-oncogene. The idea was that certain normal genes in cells such as the normal src gene could be changed or mutated to become lethal oncogenes and that cancers could become dependent on oncogenes for their survival.

The Rous virus now had a basic molecular explanation. The cause of the crisis in the henhouse had been determined. And a huge step had been taken in cancer genetics. If the protein product of a single gene could cause and maintain cancer, finding a drug that would inhibit that protein's function and cure the cancer should be possible.

Toward that end, investigators had to do more research. By the early 1980s, several laboratories had demonstrated that the src proto-oncogene encodes a normal enzyme that transfers signals through a chain of proteins that end within the cell nucleus. Those signals control the expression of genes regulating cell division and other critical functions within the cell. Fully functional tyrosine kinases—the Greek-based name for these enzymes—contribute to a network of hundreds of signaling proteins that work together to regulate cell division, normal cell death, and the functional destiny of cells. But if a mutation of the src proto-oncogene disrupts the amino acid sequence of the src tyrosine kinase protein, then the protein can become hyperactive. By passing too many signals through the kinase chain to the cell's nucleus, the abnormal protein, now an oncoprotein, causes rapid-fire cell division and cell growth—that is, cancer.

Nineteen years after beginning his collaboration with Varmus, Bishop reported in his Nobel lecture that twenty-five oncogenes had been detected worldwide. Two of these, abl and kit, have turned out to play key roles in Ken's cancer. Kit played the more essential role in generating the GIST tumor that almost killed Ken.

The kit oncogene received its name for a simple reason: it was first discovered in kittens burdened by an RNA tumor virus that causes leukemia in cats and kittens. Investigators found that an RNA tumor virus had stolen a normal proto-oncogene from cat cells and then mutated it to become an oncogene. Other research showed that normal kit proto-oncogene is not restricted to cats; it exists in all mammalian cells, including those of humans.

Normal kit protein, the product of the kit proto-oncogene, turned out to be a tyrosine kinase, with one difference from either the src or the abl proteins. The kit protein pushes its head through the cell membrane and waves it in the fluid surrounding the cell. The rest of the protein, including its signaling tyrosine, lies in the body of the cell, waiting to pass signals when an external protein latches onto and combines tightly with the waving head.

This kind of tyrosine kinase, known as a *receptor* tyrosine kinase, is particularly useful in the development and proliferation of cells during the maturation of a fetus. Specific proteins in fluids around fetal cells that bind to receptor tyrosine kinases can start selected populations of fetal cells to divide and differentiate in order to become organs or parts of organs. Researchers have found that mice lacking essential receptor tyrosine kinases like kit or one of the specific binding proteins have different congenital abnormalities ranging from anemia and hair color loss to defective organs.

The understanding of kit's usual role in the body started with work back in the late nineteenth century when the Spanish neuroanatomist Ramón y Cajal explored the neural cells of the gastrointestinal tract. Cajal, who went on to receive a 1906 Nobel Prize for enormous contributions to neuroanatomy, had become fascinated by a rather homely mystery. As we sit enjoying a meal, we may feel the rumble of gas in our intestines. The noise signals that the bowel is doing its job—moving digested food and its accompanying gas from intake (mouth) to exit (the other end). Wavelike contractions that take place within the intestine in a synchronized manner called peristalsis regularly move the bowel contents along. Cajal wanted to know how the muscle of the bowel receives instructions to contract in this way.

The answer involved recognizing that a layer of bowel tissue contains a complex network of nervelike cells. The cells—now named for Cajal—are large and have multiple short extensions that protrude from their outer walls. The extensions of one such cell wrap around those of neighboring Cajal cells, in turn forming an ideal structure for passing along signals. Since the extensions also burrow into and connect with bowel muscles, a signal originating in a distant Cajal cell can lead to a particular segment of the bowel muscle contracting. (Without the nervelike Cajal cells, peristalsis would cease and we would be subjected to even more advertisements on television about constipation.)

Despite Cajal's elegant anatomical description of the cells named for him, proof that they actually control peristalsis did not emerge until 1995. In that year, Alan Bernstein—the current president of the Canadian Institutes of Health Research—reported that mice born without a functioning kit gene have plenty of trouble. Such unfortunate mice cannot produce the kit receptor tyrosine kinase. Bernstein had known for years that they have small eyes, abnormal coat color, and poor sperm and blood cell production. But in 1995 he observed that the mice are also chronically constipated. What defines a happy mouse is one that drops stool all over the place as it frisks around. But these mice are sluggish and unhappy; some can go days without a stool drop. They are very deficient in Cajal cells, and the few Cajal cells in their intestines lack the kit protein. Clearly, Cajal cells do drive peristalsis, and those cells cannot develop unless they are well endowed with kit.

Three years later, pathologists working in Sweden applied Bernstein's mouse studies to human cancer. Ken's tumor and others like it had originally been given a vague descriptive name because no one actually knew its cell of origin. The Swedish pathologists, suspecting Cajal cell origin, used a special stain for kit protein and found that the tumor cells stained heavily. They concluded that GISTs must arise from a cancerous Cajal cell.

One more step was necessary. Working half a world apart one year after Ken's diagnosis, Yukihiko Kitamura, a pathologist then at the Osaka University School of Medicine in Japan, and a team that included Marcia Lux, a Harvard medical student, and Jonathan Fletcher, a pathologist at the Brigham and Women's Hospital in Boston, published startling reports. They found that malignant Cajal cells in GISTs are loaded with excessive kit activity, and at least one of the two kit genes in the tumor is mutated. Kitamura had previously described rare families with inherited GISTs. In such families, the germ cells (eggs or sperm) also carried mutations in the kit gene.

Although the *amount* of kit protein in GIST cells is normal, its *activity* is enormous. Acquired GIST comes about when one of the millions of Cajal cells in the bowel suffers a mutation in one kit gene, so it produces an oncoprotein that stays active continuously. In perfect oncoprotein form, it then ceaselessly passes signals to the cell's nucleus telling it to divide. Overwhelmed, the nucleus divides and replicates rapidly, as do its daughter cells and those of future generations. The signals also enhance the cells' survival. A large tumor forms.

That is just what happened to Ken. The multiplying and long-lived Cajal cells, driven by mutant kit, eventually created a grapefruit-size mass in his intestine. As the mass enlarged, further changes occurred in some of the cancer cells: Their chromosomes broke and rearranged themselves, creating mutations in genes other than kit. The multiple mutations added fuel to the fire of unrestricted growth.

When the size of Ken's tumor reached a critical point, the cells in the middle of the cancerous mass could not receive enough blood to sustain them. As they died, they released proteins that circulated in the blood, traveled to the liver, and stimulated the liver to release the protein that causes storage cells to bind up iron and take it out of circulation. The captured iron could not become part of developing red blood cells, which caused Ken to become anemic and fooled his specialist into believing he was iron deficient. No wonder the blood transfusions didn't work.

The cancerous cells kept growing on the outside of the tumor and dying within it. Some virtually obliterated a small segment of Ken's intestinal wall. Finally, his intestinal contents spilled out and catastrophe ensued. Then it was up to Demetri to find a treatment to kill the multiple GIST tumors that would surely grow in Ken's abdomen.

By the time I met Ken, Demetri had already directed his new patient's curious mind to a trove of information about the treatment he would receive and the various approaches Demetri would take to determine the extent, if any, of his recurrent disease. Demetri needed to educate Ken carefully because his treatment plan was not standard. Not many patients with GIST also have a ruptured small intestine. The process of obtaining useful informed consent would require plenty of patient education. Much of the education would center on the influence of particular genes on his cancer and the smart drugs that would be used to destroy it.

The discovery of the smart drug for Ken had begun more than forty years before he had met Demetri. In 1960, the genetics laboratory of Peter Nowell and David Hungerford at the University of Pennsylvania had adopted what was then a new method for examining the chromosomes of cancer cells that had been induced to grow in a plastic or glass dish. They looked down their microscopes at the twenty-two pairs of chromosomes of the blood cells of patients with the rare leukemia called chronic myelogenous leukemia (CML) and saw something remarkable. They were all normal except that in every leukemic cell of every patient, one of the pair of chromosome 22s (small chromosomes to begin with) was even shorter than its small partner. For Nowell and Hungerford, the appearance of the chromosomes, particularly the easily discernible, small 22 that became known as the Philadelphia chromosome, provided an important diagnostic test for CML. They published the finding immediately. Now, they thought, CML could be diagnosed unequivocally.

That observation, startling at the time, was the beginning of the development of an effective treatment for Ken. Thirteen years later, Janet Rowley, a geneticist at the University of Chicago, looked even more carefully at the blood cells of patients with CML and noticed that one of the pair of the larger chromosome 9s seemed longer than its partner. Within the next three decades, other scientists, particularly David Baltimore and Owen Witte at MIT, confirmed that the Philadelphia chromosome and the slightly longer chromosome 9 are due to breaks near the middle of chromosome 22 and at the tip of chromosome 9. The large broken-off piece of chromosome 22 is transferred to the breakpoint at the tip of the fractured chromosome 9, making it longer than normal. In exchange, a very small fragment of the broken-off chromosome 9 is transferred to the breakpoint on the fractured chromosome 22, leaving it considerably shorter than normal. This kind of exchange is called a reciprocal translocation as also described in Mario's story.

All of this would be interesting biology and nothing more if it were not for the remarkable fact that the translocation that produces the Philadelphia chromosome is responsible for leukemia. Reciprocal translocations probably occur in dividing cells frequently. After all, every time a cell divides, twenty-two pairs of chromosomes and two sex-determining chromosomes line themselves up, duplicate, and dump themselves properly in the nuclei of dividing cells. There have to be occasional errors in such a complex process. That a few errors such as translocations occur during cell division in several of the swarm of cells that are dividing in us every day is not at all surprising. Fortunately, the cells that bear such errors usually die, so we never see them. But some translocations—such as happened in Mario's MLL or that which causes the Philadelphia chromosome—favor a cell for survival. And the progeny of such survival-advantaged cells with "favorable" translocations appropriate the bone marrow.

In the case of CML, the reason for the takeover is now readily explained. Included in the tip of chromosome 9 that is transferred to chromosome 22 is the normal tyrosine kinase gene known as c-abl. It produces one of the more than five hundred enzyme proteins called kinases that normally work quietly together to regulate the growth of cells. CML is due to a single event in one bone marrow cell. In that cell, an innocent c-abl gene, yanked from its normal resting place on chromosome 9, is plastered onto the remaining bit of a broken chromosome 22 (the Philadelphia chromosome) at a DNA site called bcr (breakpoint cluster region).

While the broken-off piece of chromosome 22 that ends up pasted onto the remaining tip of chromosome 9 can be forgotten, the forced union of bcr DNA with abl DNA on the Philadelphia chromosome forms an abnormal gene that produces a new and much longer fusion protein called bcr-abl. That fusion protein, like the mutated kit protein that attacked Ken, has much more tyrosine kinase activity. It is an oncoprotein like src, and the bcr-abl DNA is an oncogene. The reciprocal translocation transforms a formerly innocent c-abl into a monster. The constant signaling from the bcr-abl tyrosine kinase becomes a driving force that demands cell growth. It influences the bone marrow cell in which the translocation occurs to divide and avoid the death pathway. The result is chronic myelogenous leukemia. Unlike the translocation that occurred in Mario's bone marrow and forced activation of MLL, the bcr-abl translocation does not require a second "hit" to initiate leukemia. George Daley, a young medical student in David Baltimore's laboratory at MIT, showed in 1990 that bcr-abl can cause leukemia by itself just as activated kit can itself force a Cajal cell to form a gastrointestinal stromal tumor.

Since the discovery of the Philadelphia chromosome, nearly all leukemias, including Mario's MLL leukemia, have been shown to be due in part to reciprocal translocations; tyrosine kinases have been demonstrated to play a role in causing GIST sarcomas, breast, colon, and thyroid cancers, as well as some leukemias. Researchers have also found that many types of cancer develop from mutations of other growth-promoting or death pathway–controlling genes. Modern cancer genetics has grown out of one simple observation made by three investigators peering down a microscope at the blood cell chromosomes in a rare leukemia.

Effective treatment for Ken emerged from an initial attack on the bcr-abl oncoprotein. The abl tyrosine kinase gene in its rightful location on chromosome 9 is, like the src tyrosine kinase that intrigued Michael Bishop and Harold Varmus, one of many signaling kinase genes in cells. A kinase protein passes growth signals along the cell-signaling network by moving high-energy phosphorus molecules from one protein to another, just as relays pass messages along phone lines. The abl gene, when normally present on chromosome 9, is almost always quiet and cooperative, switching on and off when required, but when it is fused to bcr DNA on chromosome 22, the fusion keeps the abl kinase in the "on" position. The result is a surfeit of abl kinase activity in the cell. The excess kinase activity bursts out of the confines of the signaling controls · of the cell and causes unbridled growth or cancer. To pursue the phone analogy, the line is always open.

There matters stood for a while as the information percolated through the scientific and pharmaceutical company communities. Alex Matter, then a science leader at Ciba-Geigy Pharmaceuticals in Switzerland, is a bright man who reads omnivorously. Most of the information about src and abl was available to him when he decided to launch a major research effort in the 1980s to find drugs that would inhibit tyrosine kinases in human cancers. But he needed a model screening system with which he could efficiently test the huge libraries of small molecules that Ciba-Geigy had in its secret possession. He found the major tools for his screening system at Dana-Farber Cancer Institute in the laboratories of Tom Roberts and Chuck Stiles. Their collaboration rapidly led to the first antikinase therapy for fighting cancer.

Roberts and a fledgling clinical fellow, Brian Druker, provided Matter and his team at Ciba-Geigy (which would become Novartis in 1996 after Sandoz Pharmaceuticals merged with Ciba-Geigy) with a screening test that detects drugs active against tyrosine kinase proteins. Together they produced a monoclonal antibody called 4G10 that detects tyrosine when a molecule of phosphorus is bound to it. The antibody would therefore detect an activated tyrosine kinase, and it could be used in a screen to find drugs that inhibit the process. Stiles provided a precious cell line that heavily expressed a tyrosine kinase known as PDGFR.

Activated abl, PDGFR, or kit have similar functions and modes of action—they send signals to the nucleus of cells to instruct them to divide, and they do so when a molecule of ATP (the energizer of the cell) bearing a "hot coal" of high-energy phosphorus pops into its special pouch in either protein. Resting there, ATP hands the "hot coal" to a nearby tyrosine, an amino acid in close proximity to the pouch. The transfer of the "hot coal" to tyrosine starts a stream of *divide now* signals to the nucleus through multiple protein kinase connections.

The 4G10 antibody and the cell line allowed Matter and his colleagues to detect any drug blocking the capacity of ATP and a tyrosine kinase like PDGFR, abl, or kit to add a phosphorus to tyrosine. Thus armed, Matter's team screened thousands of small molecules for their ability to block the binding of ATP in the pouch of the PDGFR tyrosine kinase protein. Such small molecules, they reasoned, might act as effective drugs that could block kinase-signaled cell division and thereby arrest cancer. The researchers would have to be lucky, of course. They had a haystack of small molecules in which they would have to find one or two needles—drugs that would be readily absorbed in the gastrointestinal tract, penetrate cell membranes, block the ATP-binding pouch in the target tyrosine kinases, have very low toxicity, and be reasonably specific for the target tyrosine kinase.

Incredibly, the investigators went on to find several needles: three compounds out of the many thousands that they screened seemed to work. One of them, with the code name STI-571 (signal transduction inhibitor 571), was particularly effective. It was soon to be named Gleevec. The next question was more complicated: What should Ciba-Geigy do with the drug? Serendipity came to the rescue.

In 1989, when Druker was starting his research career in the Roberts laboratory, he was well aware of chronic myelogenous leukemia because he had taken care of patients with the disease. He knew it was caused by a translocation that mutates the abl tyrosine kinase and makes it hyperactive. Immediately upon entering the laboratory, he learned of Matter's discovery of STI-571 and the inhibition of PDGFR. Druker asked a simple question: Could STI-571 also inhibit bcr-abl and thereby attack CML cells? He set about to convince Matter to develop STI-571 to treat CML.

Persuading Matter was relatively easy, but Druker found that purveying the notion to the skeptical drug company was a very tough sell. Matter's superiors in the business office at Ciba-Geigy (Novartis) were not impressed. They couldn't see how all the expensive research could translate into an effective drug for cancer treatment, especially for a relatively uncommon cancer. (At most, CML afflicts perhaps twenty thousand patients per year in the United States.) And the company had already decided to see whether the drug might prevent coronary artery grafts from narrowing by inhibiting PDGFR, which probably plays a role in that complication. Furthermore, at the time, no clear evidence existed to prove that overactive tyrosine kinases cause common human cancers.

The development of a new drug is hugely expensive. Millions must be spent on toxicity trials in animals and in toxicity and early efficacy trials in people. Plus, most drugs fail—and they tend to do so after much money has been spent on developing them. Ciba-Geigy (Novartis) would do far better by investing in making a copycat drug or creating something for big-market problems such as coronary narrowing, pimples, hair loss, or limp erections.

In order to test STI-571 in CML, the company would have to make enough of the experimental drug to go beyond the screening that it had pursued with the test provided by Roberts, Druker, and Stiles. That would cost money and use up the precious time of medicinal chemists who could be working on problems much more common than CML. But Druker, who had just moved to a new laboratory at the Oregon Health and Sciences University, persisted. Matter finally gave him a small supply of STI-571 for laboratory studies.

It worked—tremendously! In the laboratory, it killed CML cells that Druker had been given by Jim Griffin, one of his mentors at Dana-Farber. Druker began to beat the drum ceaselessly on Matter, imploring him to persuade Novartis to make enough of the drug for a phase 1 clinical trial.

Druker won. The trial proved hugely successful. CML patients went into remission with little or no toxicity, and Novartis received the best publicity any big pharmaceutical company had gained for several years.

Sidney Farber's magic bullet seemed to have arrived. Druker and the Novartis team received one prize after another. Sadly, Roberts and Stiles were barely noticed, but their work had established an approach to an effective treatment for thousands of leukemia patients and would soon translate into a new treatment for Ken and many others like him.

# CHAPTER EIGHTEEN

# Triumph and Tragedy

W hen I first met George Demetri at Dana-Farber Cancer Institute, I immediately thought he was a terrific physician investigator.

"I've been involved with cancer from the time I was a kid," Demetri told me. "There was always somebody in my family who had cancer. As a child growing up and seeing the adults around me getting radiation and all the attendant side effects, and chemotherapy and all those side effects, . . . I always wanted to see if I could . . . help make the therapies easier and better in the future."

The 1980s were disappointing for Demetri and the few clever experimental oncologists like him. There were new chemotherapeutic drugs and better supportive therapies, but the survival of people with some of the most common cancers—colon, lung, advanced breast, and prostate—improved only slightly during that time.

Demetri understood that a new approach was badly needed. He decided to focus his efforts on sarcomas because he worried that the more common kinds of tumors (the epithelial cancers including breast, colon, lung, and prostate) might not be the best first choice for investigation. The extensive chromosome damage from the start in common cancers suggested they might have so many growth gene abnormalities that finding one Achilles' heel might be very unlikely.

The chromosomes of sarcomas are often abnormal, but their abnormalities begin as relatively simpler changes. Demetri reasoned that if sarcomas could be detected early, they might be susceptible to smart drugs. He decided to focus on GIST.

Fortunately, a Japanese postdoctoral fellow—in the same laboratory as Demetri—had once worked in Kitamura's group in Osaka. He told

186

Demetri of the discovery of high kit activity in GIST cells. Excitedly, Demetri told the sarcoma group of surgeons, oncologists, and pathologists about the Osaka findings. These were old hat to a sarcoma group member, Jonathan Fletcher, the pathologist at the Brigham and Women's Hospital, who had observed the same results. It was clear to Demetri that the Kitamura and Fletcher findings blew the lid off of GIST. The increased kit activity was due to very small mutations in at least one copy of the kit gene in the tumor, a mutation that held ATP in its pocket or pouch in the protein and thereby maintained the enzyme in the "on" position. But how could the hyperactivity of kit be shut down?

The potential for success in the treatment of GIST received a huge break in 1999 when Demetri happened to talk to his former DFCI colleague, Druker, and asked Druker whether STI-571 (Gleevec) shut down tyrosine kinases other than abl. The answer was straightforward: the drug also shuts down kit.

Demetri immediately arranged a collaboration with Druker and David Tuveson, another young investigator at Dana-Farber and MIT, to determine whether Gleevec would kill GIST cells in a culture dish. The answer was strongly positive. Clearly, the mutant kit tyrosine kinase had established a strong antideath signal in GIST cells. When exposed to Gleevec, they went right down the death pathway. When ATP was forced out of the pocket in the protein by the drug and the continuous kit signal was thus blocked, the cells had no choice but to die.

Demetri still recounts the story with excitement. "I can't imagine a kinder or gentler way of killing cancer cells without injuring a patient. Why kill normal cells and hope that you happen to have a lot of the cancer cells in your field of treatment? Why pummel the patient with toxic chemotherapy? Why not just give a drug that helps the body get rid of mutated cells? . . . I wanted to start a trial of Gleevec immediately in gastrointestinal stromal tumors."

So as Druker had done before him, Demetri began a campaign to persuade Novartis to provide Gleevec for the treatment of GIST. He recalled, "Every CML patient in North America wanted the drug and they wanted it yesterday. They were literally e-mailing and protesting to Novartis that they needed to get the drug, and they needed to get it now. And Novartis, to their credit, wanted to respond, but they had not yet manufactured enough of the drug. So they were very limited on how much they would give out for exploratory studies like ours."

The story behind Novartis's decision is striking. It involves both international cooperation among scientists and a study of just one patient.

A Finnish physician had a patient with multiple GIST tumors in her abdomen. The physician had heard of Demetri's interest in Gleevec and e-mailed Demetri with a description of his patient. Demetri informed the physician that he was awaiting a decision by Novartis to make more of the drug for GIST patients. However, it turned out that the Novartis operating company for Scandinavia had a reasonable supply of Gleevec and made it available. The patient was investigated with a positron emission tomography (PET) scan utilizing radioactive sugar before and after one month of treatment. The uptake of sugar by a tumor tells whether it is living or dead. The results showed that the tumors avidly consumed sugar before treatment but did not consume it after Gleevec—they were dead. CAT scans showed that they were shrinking. "Nobody had ever seen anything like this," exulted Demetri. "And she had no side effects of any note."

The central management of Novartis was also impressed. They made Gleevec available to Demetri for what was to be a small clinical trial but turned out to be quite large. Patients with GIST began to appear from everywhere. Now that physicians knew of an effective treatment, they began to refer their patients. GIST turned out to be much more common than Demetri and his colleagues had ever believed; as common as childhood leukemia, with probably five thousand new cases occurring every year in the United States.

Demetri began to use PET scanning to monitor the responses in all of his patients. He found that securing appointments for a scan wasn't always easy because only one machine was available to him and it was heavily booked. The situation resulted in a second remarkable finding.

In one patient, Demetri organized a pretreatment PET scan that demonstrated a large GIST and several smaller tumors that were avidly consuming sugar and therefore growing. He wanted to repeat the scan after a week of treatment, but the PET scan office could only offer him a second scan one day after the first dose of Gleevec. The rest of the week was completely booked, so Demetri took the appointment. To his amazement, the repeat scan showed absolutely no sugar uptake. The scan was completely normal: one dose of Gleevec had killed the cancer cells in just one day. This showed that GISTs may be wildly aggressive and unstoppable by carpet-bombing chemotherapy, but their Achilles' heel is their dependence on kit for survival. Neither Demetri nor anyone else had ever seen a solid tumor stopped in its tracks by a single dose of any therapy.

The case offered proof that a concerted search for the pathways adopted by cancer cells to survive and a further search for smart drugs to block those pathways could be highly productive. It would lead to a sea change in cancer therapy.

The majority of the patients responded to Gleevec, although some were slower to respond than others. Eventually, with the laboratory support of Jonathan Fletcher in Boston and Mike Heinrich in Brian Druker's laboratory in Oregon, George Demetri determined that the location of the mutation in the DNA sequence of a GIST-associated kit gene strongly influenced the quality and durability of response to the drug. The same team found that a minority of GISTs are caused by similar mutations in a nearby gene, the platelet-derived growth factor receptor (PDGFR). Gleevec also blocked the signaling activity of the mutant PDGFR gene and controlled some of the GIST tumors that depended on the product of that gene.

The most remarkable fact was that the treatment was only minimally toxic. Mild fluid retention, stomach distress, and some reduction in blood cell counts were the usual side effects. The complications of the treatment were acceptable because normal cells do not absolutely depend on kit or PDGFR for their survival: they enjoy a more complex interaction of signaling proteins that govern their growth. Only GISTs absolutely require mutant kit and/or PDGFR.

As word spread, Novartis's ability to supply Gleevec became strained. The company and Demetri had planned to study thirty patients in three years. The first thirty arrived in just about one month. That made sense, since Druker's experience of leukemia had made the cover of *Time* magazine. And one of Demetri's former nurse practitioners was an Internet hobbyist who built Demetri a Web site called www.sarcoma.net. The size of his study doubled and doubled again.

But there was a downside. Most patients with CML or GIST slowly but surely develop resistance to Gleevec. Single-agent chemotherapy is almost always associated with the development of a resistant population of cancer cells that find a way to avoid the action of the drug. The resistance to Gleevec by GIST cells has proven particularly devilish. The pocket or pouch in the kit tyrosine kinase molecule in which the drug sits is lined with amino acids, the building blocks of proteins. If one of them is changed by mutation, the drug may no longer fit in the pocket and therefore fails to function. If the drug cannot get into the pocket, ATP can slide in: the kit hypersignaling starts anew. When that happens, the drug is rendered ineffectual.

A pocket amino acid mutation may occur secondary to the pressure of the drug itself. But Charles Sawyers, an investigator at the University of California in Los Angeles, has evidence that a very rare population of CML cells might contain a pocket mutation before Gleevec treatment begins. Such cells become the dominant population when the sensitive CML cells are killed. That may well happen in GIST.

On the bright side, investigators have found that resistance-provoking second mutations do not, however, necessarily spell doom for smart drug therapy. Sugen (now owned by Pfizer), Novartis, and Bristol-Meyers Squibb have fashioned other smart drugs to fit the mutated pouch. In the summer of 2004, Charles Sawyers reported that a new Bristol-Meyers Squibb drug, BMS-354825, or dasatinib, is twice as potent as Gleevec (imatinib) and kills chronic myelogenous leukemia cells that have pouch mutations in their abl genes and are therefore resistant to Gleevec. A second approach is to add standard chemotherapy to the smart drug. Even if the carpet bombers do not work alone, they may be synergistic when added to Gleevec.

Finally, researchers can take advantage of the fact that the kit signal passes through many relay stations on its way to the nucleus. Each of the relay stations is governed by a signal protein (often a kinase) produced by an independent gene. Drugs can be made that would attack the relay proteins, thereby targeting several key steps simultaneously in a signaling cascade that starts with kit or PDGFR and ends with growth and antideath signals in the cell nucleus. Accordingly, in 2002, Demetri started trying to combat drug resistance by working with new combinations of smart drugs. Given enough time, he thought he would find the right formula.

Scores of patients with GISTs and other sarcomas continued to make their way to Demetri. Among them was Ken, who knew that his chances of developing recurrent and multiple GIST tumors were life-threateningly high. He arrived in Demetri's clinic in November 1999 feeling much better but worried that he would soon have a recurrence. Demetri agreed that he probably would. "He said to me [that] I'd be dealing with it again," Ken recalled. "He said, 'I can't tell you when, but we'll monitor you, we'll keep an eye on it. We know what we're looking at; we know what we're looking for.'"

Ken left with a sense of hope. "The first medicine that this hospital gave me was hope," he commented as he spoke with me one day at Dana-Farber. Referring to Demetri, he added, "There was something about him that just exuded confidence, but the confidence was based in real knowledge."

Ken went on. "George Demetri said, 'You're here at the perfect point in history. There's a tremendous amount of work going on in this field right now. You've got a cancer that we know a lot about genetically, and we're going to know more about it as we go down the road together.' I think that's all come to fruition. So it wasn't just hope, it was a promise kept. And he's done that, and in spades. He's been a remarkable man."

In June 2000, a PET scan showed that Ken had at least forty small GIST tumors and four larger ones. They had each arisen from one of the cells that had spewed out of the original tumor and had lodged undetected in separate crevices throughout his abdomen. Ken needed treatment, but Gleevec had not yet been cleared for use in GIST.

"George tried me on an experimental drug called ET-743—to no avail," Ken pointed out. "It had no effect on me. He just kept smiling and saying, 'Don't worry. We've got this thing coming along called STI-571 (Gleevec),' which was for the longest time going to be my license plate. He said, 'We've got that thing coming; it looks very good. The mice seem to love it'—or whatever. So we were patient, and fortunately nothing was pressing a major organ. He started me on the Gleevec in July of 2000. It was almost exactly a year to the day that the tumor had burst into my belly.

"Within two weeks, all the tumors in my belly were cold (meaning that the PET scan showed no uptake of sugar), which I never expected. I expected five or ten percent or some number to be handed to me like that. And when he came inside and said, 'Your whole scan is cold,' I think it was just one of the happiest days of my life."

Some weeks later, a CT scan of Ken's belly found that the tumors were shrinking. Ken became a poster boy for Gleevec and the treatment of GIST for two years, from 2000 to 2002. He spoke on the radio as a cancer survivor, appeared on a cancer special that played on the HBO television channel, and was featured in a long *New York Times* article on new anticancer drugs.

But Ken was warned that he would encounter more difficulty. Demetri knew that the emergence of resistance is virtually the rule in single-agent chemotherapy and assumed the treatment with Gleevec would lead to a similar situation. In July 2002, a routine PET scan showed that a few of Ken's tumors were now consuming sugar. They were growing very slowly, not yet impinging on any vital organs, but they needed to be treated.

Ken became a subject of new clinical trials focusing on other smart-drug possibilities. Initially, Demetri did not have anything in his pocket that had the promise of Gleevec. In early 2002, the smart drug SU11248 (sunitinib) manufactured by Sugen Pharmaceuticals (now part of Pfizer) became available to Demetri for a limited trial two years before its application in larger trials. The drug had been designed to overcome resistance to Gleevec in chronic myelogenous leukemia, but laboratory studies showed that it also inhibited the activity of other tyrosine kinases such as kit. Demetri decided to ask Ken to try the drug, and Ken agreed. Unfortunately, from 2002 to 2004, little happened with sunitinib or other drugs Demetri tried. Although the tumors occasionally regressed or became much colder on the PET scan, subsequently they would slowly recover. Then Ken would receive another combination of drugs or a single agent.

Ken maintained a strong, positive attitude about the situation. "I don't believe in that old saw 'when life gives you lemons, make lemonade,'" he told me. "I believe when life gives you lemons, it's lemon season—enjoy them. Some day it's going to give you cherries or whatever else, but enjoy them—it's lemon season [now]. And if you can smile with a lemon, the rest of it's downhill; the rest of it's just going to happen.

"I've developed this philosophy because I've read my whole life," Ken continued. "I've tried to figure out the meaning of life since I was ten years old. I've always been fascinated with the question, and it's been the point of my existence to answer it. Sometime around my fortieth birthday, I realized I was asking the wrong question. It's not, 'What's the meaning of life in general?' but, 'What's the meaning of my life?'"

Ken found answers from reading Viktor Frankel's book *Man's Search for Meaning*. He was influenced by the fact that Frankel had "survived Auschwitz and came out with a philosophy of life that means something to me. We each have to find that meaning in our life. Maybe my meaning is to be a compass needle that points to Demetri. . . . Maybe I'm here to say to another confused and frightened cancer patient, 'Look, if you don't get anything out of Ken's story, at least go to a cancer hospital with experts and get that second opinion. Demand that second opinion; get the experts, get the cutting-edge technology available to you.' If that's all my cancer does for me, that's okay. My life will be worthwhile if I have helped someone else."

Though Ken followed instructions to the letter and faithfully complied with all of Demetri's ideas, the results were disappointing. His tumors continued to grow slowly and inexorably as the dose was escalated. The trial had to be considered a failure for him. Both Demetri and Ken were bitterly disappointed, but Demetri maintained an optimistic stance. The Bristol-Meyers Squibb drug called dasatinib was now ready for clinical trials. This was the drug that Charles Sawyers had shown to be capable of overcoming Gleevec resistance in chronic myelogenous leukemia and later shown to be active as well in many Gleevec-resistant GIST cells. It seemed to offer a perfect solution for Ken. He consented to join a dose escalation trial in the summer of 2004 and became the first solid tumor patient in the world to receive the new drug.

Though Demetri firmly believed that the new smart drug would control the growth of Ken's tumor, the course of the trial was both disappointing and discouraging. There were three immediate difficulties. The first related to the awkwardness of the measurement of response in a patient with multiple tumors even by PET scan. A PET scan image of Ken's abdomen revealed that some of his more than forty tumors took up radioactive glucose whereas others did not. Some were larger by MRI and some were smaller. A system of measurement had to be devised that would provide some quantitative assessment of tumor growth, but the results could be variable from day to day. Only measurements of trends over a prolonged time course could provide accurate data.

The second difficulty was related to the first. Because serial measurements were required to determine efficacy, the number of days required at each dose was necessarily very high. Each dose required a commitment of two months before the patient could move to the next dose, and the actual increments in dose were very small. Months could drift by with no evidence of any efficacy.

The third and most serious difficulty was a toxic side effect at higher doses. The phase 1 trial featured dose escalation in an effort to determine toxicity. Effectiveness would also be measured, but the major goal of the trial was the determination of a tolerable dose. When that dose was found, a subsequent phase 2 trial would provide a better understanding of efficacy.

Unfortunately, Ken began to experience serious psychiatric problems at the higher doses, and only at those doses was there any evidence, however uncertain, that the drug was shutting down the ability of his tumor to consume glucose. As the dose of drug was slowly increased, Ken began to become increasingly listless. His appetite declined, and his upbeat personality became flat and unemotional. In addition, he had persistent abdominal pain that he knew must be due to one or more tumors pressing on a nerve in his belly. He did not want to give up on dasatinib because he and Demetri had invested so much hope in it, but his pain and his obvious depression began to consume most of his waking hours. And there was no evidence that the drug was controlling the growth of his tumors.

Before long, Ken was in a terrible mental state. He didn't want to get out of bed in the morning, an unheard-of characteristic for him. He slept as much as possible during the day and was restless and sleepless at night. Black thoughts began to preoccupy him. He thought of suicide.

Demetri sought an opinion from a psychiatrist, who immediately diagnosed acute depression. The question that had to be faced was very complex. Was the depression due to the drug or due to abdominal pain and severe discouragement because Ken had expected the drug to help? There was no obvious way to tell the difference. There are no tests that distinguish drug-induced symptoms from endogenous psychiatric symptoms.

No matter how "smart" a drug may be, all drugs are essentially poisons that interrupt metabolic pathways. The purpose of a phase 1 clinical trial is to find a dose at which toxicity occurs with the hope that therapeutic benefit is achieved at a lower dose. The therapeutic-to-toxic dose ratio of a drug is calculated by dividing the dose that achieves a favorable response by the dose that causes toxic side effects. The lower that ratio, the better the drug. But the ratio must be carefully described. Many forms of toxicity are of little consequence, and patients usually tolerate them very well. Gleevec is such a drug. It does cause side effects, but almost all patients can live quite comfortably with the symptoms.

Aspirin, considered safe by almost everyone, is actually a very dangerous drug when examined solely from the point of view of its therapeutic-to-toxic ratio. It's therapeutic intent is to relieve aches and pain and lower body temperature, but at any dose that achieves those therapeutic benefits, the drug severely inhibits blood platelet function and is apt to cause dangerous bleeding. In fact, the toxic dose is far lower than the therapeutic dose. The therapeutic-to-toxic ratio is infinitely high. Ironically, this terrible therapeutic-to-toxic ratio has been used for a secondary and much more valuable therapeutic benefit. Regular but small doses of aspirin are taken with excellent effect by millions to delay the onset of coronary artery disease. So rigid interpretation of phase 1 clinical trials by drug regulators such as the Food and Drug Administration (FDA) would be counterproductive and defeating for the very patients who are the beneficiaries of FDA efforts—if the agency is not crippled by political zealots in the White House.

There is a further and entirely unpredictable aspect of the therapeutic-to-toxic dose ratio that may or may not be detected in a phase 1 clinical trial unless it involves a large number of patients. Though almost all individuals have the same compliment of twenty thousand to twenty-five thousand genes, there may be many variations of genes that affect the absorption of a drug from the gastrointestinal tract, its clearance from the circulation, its breakdown in the liver, its excretion in the bile or in the urine, and its penetration of organs such as the brain. Such genetic variations may lead to unique drug reactions that are entirely unexpected and may occur without warning. These so-called idiosyncratic reactions are often unrelated to dose, and they may produce very severe toxic side effects. An entire field of medicine called pharmacogenetics has been developed to find ways to detect susceptible patients before reactions occur.

Severe depression is not a common manifestation of dasatinib toxicity. But Demetri had to conclude that it might have penetrated Ken's brain in some unique way and damaged the function of the delicate network of nerves that control emotion. Demetri had no choice. In late February 2005, he stopped the drug to see what would happen to Ken's badly depressed psyche.

Within a few days, Demetri's decision was rewarded. Ken was a new man. His depression lifted, his suicidal ideas vanished, and despite his abdominal pain, his optimistic approach to life returned. Demetri then decided to pursue what some might have considered a useless gamble. He had not abandoned the idea of testing newer receptor tyrosine kinase inhibitors in Ken. Though both SU11248 and dasatinib had been failures in Ken, another even more promising kinase inhibitor produced by Novartis, AMN107 (nilotinib), was about to be released for phase 1 trials in CML patients resistant to Gleevec. Demetri unleashed a drumbeat campaign to persuade Novartis to release the new drug for a single-patient trial in Ken.

Pharmaceutical companies loathe single-patient drug trials. During the early trial stages of the development of any new drug, companies must report all adverse reactions to the FDA, and there is now pressure on companies to report all adverse reactions to the FDA throughout the life of a drug. Obviously, companies do not want to set themselves up for a regulatory nightmare. The chances of improvement of a single sick patient are small, but the chances of trouble and a complication that may or may not be due to the drug are high. An accumulation of toxic side effects in single patients from whom little useful clinical data can be obtained represents a foolish investment to any sensible pharmaceutical executive. Novartis wanted to develop nilotinib stepwise and carefully. It was designed to deal with mutations in the abl oncogene in chronic myelogenous leukemia. A single complex patient with GIST would have to come later.

From the point of view of a conservative Swiss drug company, the adverse decision came as no surprise, but Novartis had not often dealt with an investigator as persistent as Demetri. Scores of e-mails later, Novartis officials reluctantly agreed to allow Demetri to treat Ken, and Demetri immediately requested the Dana-Farber Institutional Review Board (IRB) to permit him to use the new drug immediately. To his surprise, the IRB wanted to have much more information before it would sanction the experiment. Demetri was furious when he received notice that his request for immediate use of AMN107 for Ken could not be granted without extensive review.

The life of a clinical investigator, a physician who wants to translate the fruits of biomedical science into patient care, can be discouraging. There are multiple barriers to clinical research that can create incredible delays. Arguments with pharmaceutical companies about the availability of new drugs in the development process and endless debates with IRBs about the ethics of research protocols are responsible for much of the delay.

As mentioned in Mario's story, prior to World War II and for two or three decades after the war, physicians were largely free to use their own judgment and their own ethical standards to determine the suitability of a given patient for a particular research procedure. Clinical research flourished in that unfettered period when physicians were universally trusted to do their best for their patients. But the demonic corruption of the Nazi physicians and the shocking realization that career officers of the U.S. Public Health Service had withheld penicillin from poor uneducated black citizens of Tuskegee, Alabama, who were afflicted with syphilis, destroyed that peaceful assumption. Congress heard cries for tighter regulation of clinical research. An initial trickle of rules became a torrent as more cases of research malfeasance were bruited about.

One of the best regulations was the creation of IRBs in 1979. Each grantee institution, usually an academic health center, was charged with the formation of a local IRB, a group of scientists, physicians, nurses, and local citizens whose task is to read a research proposal carefully and judge its ethical soundness. Great attention is paid to the quality of informed consent of the patients/subjects, and very close attention is also paid to the research protocol to be certain that the risk of the research does not approach or surpass its purported benefit.

Informed consent is a procedure in which the researcher or an agent of the researcher carefully explains the intended benefits and the attendant risks of a research proposal to a patient who will be the subject of that research. Urged by their apprehensive institutions to comply fully with informed consent procedures, physician scientists have gained "assistance" from institutional lawyers who help them write documents that may be sound legally but often adopt arcane language that covers all perils but is nowhere near the quality of a simple conversation between the would-be researcher and the patient. Given the inevitability of obfuscation when lawyers interject themselves between doctors and patients, it is imperative for the physician or the physician's agent to write a note in plain English in the medical record that describes the conversation between the researcher and the patient in some detail. If there is a later misunderstanding, that note may be the only useful record that defends the physician and his or her institution from a malpractice charge based on failure of informed consent. Sadly, the requirement for such a note is often honored in the breach.

Informed consent procedures are not unduly time-consuming, and they are rewarding because they offer an opportunity for the physician to have an intimate discussion with a frightened patient who may gain a lot of reassurance from the encounter. The patient's questions may also uncover some areas of confusion in the research protocol, clarification of which can help the investigator establish a better protocol or justify the one that is under discussion.

Most of the agonizing delay that results from the enforced nexus of the investigator with the IRB is derived from weaknesses in the research protocol itself. The protocol may be crystal clear to its author but may contain confusing elements to individuals who are less well versed in the science or are searching for ethical issues rather than scientific ones. Statisticians on IRBs may feel that the number of research subjects proposed for study in a protocol is too small to provide valid results. Since the ethics of research depends on an acceptable risk-to-benefit ratio, an inadequate study that cannot possibly answer a question is basically unethical.

There is a third disturbing feature of research carried out in patients or normal human subjects that has received recent public attention. Skillful research physicians may own stock in a company that makes a drug that they plan to administer to a patient or they may be paid consultants to the company or accept gifts from the company such as luxury travel. IRBs, investigative reporters, members of Congress, and most U.S. citizens find such conflicts of interest repugnant. When the events are revealed, there is usually a public outcry, and the case for clinical research is weakened. Physicians must avoid such conflicts. By entering them, they damage themselves and the research enterprise. Informing a patient of such conflicts does not solve the problem. They simply cannot happen.

In Demetri's case, the IRB wanted to be sure that a single patient study could provide useful information. Many of the members shared the skepticism of Novartis. Though Dana-Farber created that particular IRB, the members were entirely independent of the cancer center. They made up their own minds, and they were free to demand any and all corrections as they saw fit.

Seeing that a delay was inevitable, Demetri decided on a different tack. Ken had not taken any Gleevec for two years. Was it possible that the majority of his tumors had undergone enough mutations to regain sensitivity to Gleevec? On the basis of that hope, Demetri recommended a course of Gleevec for Ken.

To the delight of patient and physician, many of Ken's tumors grew cold on the PET scan after two weeks of Gleevec treatment, and they began to shrink. Clearly the cells in some of the tumors had developed enough mutations to permit access of the drug to the critical pouch in the kit protein into which ATP must fit. Once again, Gleevec blocked the function of the mutated and hyperactive kit receptor tyrosine kinase that drove Ken's tumors. Ken's abdominal pain decreased. Meanwhile, Demetri dealt with the criticism of the IRB and prepared to start Ken on Novartis's AMN107 when the tumors mutated again and became Gleevec resistant.

Ken's story is as much about new methods of monitoring tumors as it is about smart drugs to treat them. Patients like Ken have had an enormous influence on the technology of imaging of solid tumors. The PET scanner has become an expensive but absolutely necessary approach to measurement of the responses of solid tumors to treatment. No other imaging or laboratory measurement gives as much information in as short a period of time. But positron-labeled sugar, though very useful, is not an ideal detector of living cancer cells because it is not specific for cancer. Inflammatory cells that regularly surround cancer cells also eat up glucose and test positive in the PET scan. Other more cancer-specific positron-emitting agents are now in development. PET scanning will be much more accurate and specific within the next five years.

While all this progress swirled around him, Ken remained reflective and philosophical. "I'm working and I'm trying to stay interested. You certainly get distracted in a situation like this, where it's every two or three weeks there's a new protocol. By the same token, that's what I'm asked to do right now. I'm trying to do it with dignity.

"It's funny in a way. It's made me a better salesman in a sort of dark, sardonic way. Someone will say, 'No, I don't want that,' and I'll cough a little bit on the other end of the line and say, 'Sure would be nice to get an order before I meet the Big Guy!' And they'll say, 'You're sick!' But they tend to want to give me the order. Of course, it's not easy to be focused. I have to be in for checkups very frequently. So I don't have long periods when I do not think about the cancer and what is going on in me. But I always get a lift from this place. It's remarkable—the smiles, the laughter, and the encouragement. I walk in and now even the parking guys wave to me. I think they think I work here.

"Everybody's been wonderful. They've all been so supportive. They always ask how I'm doing in the protocol or ask me what protocol I am in. I'm in sales—I know how important it is and how much companies spend on training. This isn't training. This is honestly caring. They really care about me, and there's no phony smile. The more you come here, the kinder they are. I don't think there's any place better. When friends tell me about cancers in the family, I always tell them, 'Just do yourself a favor—just call, get a second opinion. If you don't like Dana-Farber, go to MD Anderson, go to Memorial in New York, go to some other reputable hospital that specializes in cancer and cancer research.'"

I asked Ken whether he thought some patients avoid cancer centers because they are afraid of the word and afraid of the finality of coming to such a center.

"Sure, it's the reality—'I really have cancer,'" he said. "I think it's also about our perennial denial of how our own book ends. I know how my book ends. I know there's an Author writing it right now. My argument with Him is what page it ends on—but not how. And it's a one-sided argument. I'm saying, 'Not page fifty-four!' He's going, 'Well, it's a mystery, my friend. At least for you.'

"But people are in such denial about it. Cancer is a disease where you're more afraid of the cure than the disease. They've seen the horror stories of chemo. They've seen the people dragging themselves across the television set and completely wiped out, and they're terrified of that. They saw Uncle Vinnie: 'Oh, his death was horrible. I'm not going to go that way.' Well, my God, you've got to try to beat the cancer as best you can, with as much dignity as you can, and not be afraid of the word *cancer*.

"There are other words to be afraid of that are more debilitating to the human spirit than cancer. Fear is one of them; to live in fear your whole life, when you know the outcome. Celebrate that as best you can. If this is going to be my last day, I want it to be a day of my authorship. It's my writing it as best I can and with dignity. You can't die with dignity if you don't live with it. So you have cancer, and you face it, and you say, 'I am going to try to hold my head up. I am going to go home tonight and cry maybe, but I'm going to try to spend twenty of these hours today with my head up'—as best I can."

I asked Ken how Peggy, who had insisted that he see George Demetri, was holding up during this long struggle.

"People meet my wife and they say 'sweet Peggy.' Peggy is this calm, gentle spirit. You would think she is Betty Crocker incarnate. She has been a tiger through this. She is my advocate and she's my guardian. She's got her moments of weakness, as I do, but we both try to do the same thing—we try to be prepared for the worst but to enjoy the best while we have the best. And she's done a great job with that.

"It's a terrible prospect to have to face the possibility of being alone. We're high school sweethearts. We dated in the eleventh grade, until Jimmy McMillan came along, and then got back together, and we got married. I've known her since I was eleven years old. She is my best friend, and to live without each other would be devastating.

"She's done her best to live this thing true to her values. I think she's done a great job on that. I owe her everything. I owe her to keep trying to win. And I will!"

But Ken's will and his upbeat philosophy could not stop the march of mutation in the kit tyrosine kinase that drove his tumor. His tumors became resistant to Gleevec once again. The Novartis drug AMN107 that was so effective in CML was without any influence on the growth of the multiple GIST tumors in Ken's belly. They grew and they impinged on the sensitive nerves in his abdomen. The pain was severe. Demetri knew that he was finally out of new tricks for his patient. He gave Ken prescriptions for pain relief and sent him home to spend his last days with his devoted Peggy. He died peacefully in the winter of 2005.

Ken was a persistent patient, and George Demetri is a persistent physician. Together they were marching down a century-old path of progress in basic biology that began with Ramón y Cajal and Peyton Rous and was broadened by Mike Bishop and Harold Varmus. That basic information was translated in the 1980s and 1990s from neuroanatomy and viruses to an understanding of the plight of constipated mice and then to the mechanism of cancer in the Cajal cells that cause gastrointestinal stromal tumors.

At about the same time, David Baltimore, George Daley, and Owen Witte plumbed the molecular depths of the Philadelphia chromosome and demonstrated that chronic myelogenous leukemia is due to hyperactivation of a gene called abl, a tyrosine kinase. Alex Matter and a team at Novartis were determined to uncover drugs that would block the hyperactivity of kinases in cancer. Charles Stiles and Tom Roberts provided Matter's team with the antibody and the target cells they needed to screen compounds that led to Gleevec, the first effective smart drug. Brian Druker had the insight and persistence to use Gleevec successfully in the treatment of chronic myelogenous leukemia and told George Demetri that the drug was also effective in the blockade of function of hyperactive kit. Demetri grabbed that information and applied it successfully in GIST. Charles Sawyers explored the molecular basis of resistance to tryrosine kinase inhibitors and showed that drugs similar to Gleevec could overcome it.

Ken was the indirect beneficiary of that one-hundred-year history. He became a vanguard of the revolution in smart-drug treatment for cancer. That a single drug could force a solid tumor to disappear without significant toxicity had not previously been observed. But Ken's story reiterates the absolute necessity for combination therapy to prevent drug resistance. That lesson was learned a half century earlier by those who attacked the then-intractable childhood leukemias. Smart drugs like Gleevec will force cancer to become a treatable chronic disease. But we need more of them and more knowledge of the pathways that cancer cells are forced to take to survive. Fortunately, progress in smart-drug development is flowing. It is not yet in full spate, but the stream of effective new smart drugs is widening.

# CHAPTER NINETEEN

# The Search for More Smart Drugs

Since the early 1980s when Robert Weinberg and Philip Leder described the importance of myc and ras in cancer, pharmaceutical companies have been busy trying to create drugs that might block the function or the production of oncoproteins and the growth-signaling circuits they activate. Drugs that inhibit myc are technically difficult to design, and progress has been slow. Ras sits in a very strategic position in cells. It is activated by signals that originate on the cell membrane, and it passes those signals on via a cascade of kinase proteins. As described in Ken's story, the cascade of kinases ultimately delivers a message to the nucleus to drive cell division and prevent cell death. So hyperactive ras, and in turn hyperactivation of the kinase cascade downstream of ras, causes cancer.

Despite a lot of effort, a good ras inhibitor has not yet been detected, so cancer researchers and pharmaceutical companies have searched for inhibitors of proteins that operate farther down the ras pathway. Some of the proteins in the ras-activated cascade have bizarre shorthand names like raf, mek, and erk. Indeed, a modestly good inhibitor of raf has very recently been made by Bayer Pharmaceuticals. It is still highly experimental. It is called Bay 43-9006 and has the chemical name sorafenib. It has a reasonable affinity or stickiness for the raf protein, though it also blocks other kinases as well, which may limit its tolerance by normal cells.

Other more selective inhibitors have been made by several additional pharmaceutical companies. According to early reports, there have been somewhat encouraging responses to the weaker Bayer drug against kidney tumors, or when it is combined with carpet-bombing chemotherapy, possibly against malignant melanoma, often an intractable malignancy that usually originates in the skin but may arise anywhere in the body. Scientists at Dana-Farber and elsewhere have clearly established a central role of raf in the growth of melanomas. More experience of better raf inhibitors is needed, but the results already provide proof that understanding the pathways that cancer cells adopt to ensure their survival and administering a drug to block that pathway will target the tumor at its very engine, in which resistance will be less likely to arise.

In another approach, reported in 2004, scientists at Hoffmann-LaRoche Laboratories have decided to attack a very common genetic problem in cancer cells: the deficiency of the sniffing protein called p53. As discussed in Joan's story, p53 is a central actor in many different cancers including breast cancer. It detects injured genes in cells and sends these cells down the one-way chute to death, as Stanley Korsmeyer discovered decades ago when he was beginning his brilliant research career at the National Cancer Institute in Bethesda, Maryland.

When p53 levels or the activity of p53 decline, cells with DNA damage often fail to die when they otherwise should do so. The activity of p53 is often decreased in epithelial cancers like breast cancer and many others either because its genes become mutated or because another protein called mdm2 is overactivated by mutation. In its overactive state, it avidly binds normal p53. As a result of the excessive binding of normal p53 by mutated mdm2, the p53 is literally taken out of cellular circulation. The captured protein loses its function.

If a drug could be found to elevate the levels of normal p53 in cancer cells, the cancer cells would die. The scientists at Hoffmann-LaRoche have found a small molecule that they call Nutlin because the laboratory is in Nutley, New Jersey. Nutlin prevents binding of normal p53 to mdm2, which causes the p53 levels in cancer cells to increase, thereby killing them. That is surely a smart anticancer compound. If proven effective in patients, it could be useful in treating many cancers.

In yet another novel approach, scientists in England have decided to attack cancers by assaulting their weaknesses rather than inhibiting their strengths (the latter exemplified by overactive tyrosine kinases such as kit in Ken's story). The weakness of many cancers lies in their defective DNA repair kits. For example, women who have inherited defective BRCA (a DNA repair gene) develop breast cancer at very high rates early in life. Those cancer cells survive only because there are secondary repair pathways in all cells that keep BRCA-deficient cells intact. In 2005, British scientists showed that inhibition of the secondary pathways with a drug selectively kills BRCA-deficient cancer cells. Clearly, the inhibitors of the secondary pathway could be made into very smart drugs for patients with breast cancer who are BRCA deficient.

Along different lines, Loren Walensky, a young physician scientist highly trained in chemistry, has developed a way to convert the small active site of large proteins into much smaller stable compounds that can be used as drugs. By doing so, he can create a small molecule that actually delivers a death signal to a cancer cell. His approach, published in 2004, is very likely to end in the production of new classes of smart drugs that initiate direct killing of cancer cells.

Some very promising smart drugs are already in the clinic. As mentioned in Joan's story, the first ones are not drugs in the sense of a pill. Instead, they are monoclonal antibodies designed to block the function of receptor tyrosine kinases that contribute to cancer cell proliferation. The main targets of such antibodies are the four-member family of receptor tyrosine kinase proteins known as epidermal growth factor receptors (EGFRs). These include Herceptin, the first smart anticancer compound to be proven clinically useful.

As also mentioned in Joan's story, Herceptin is an antibody directed against the cell surface receptor portion of a specialized protein, the product of one of the four members of the EGFR gene family. The particular member of interest is Her2/neu. That gene is overexpressed and makes too much protein in about one-quarter of patients with breast cancer. The overexpression of the gene fills the surface of the cancer cell with Her2/neu protein, a very active EGFR-type tyrosine kinase and a signaling protein like kit that sends messages to the cancer cell nucleus demanding that it divide.

Herceptin, the antibody, binds the excess protein on the cell surface and prevents it from signaling. A recently completed study of Herceptin has shown that the drug markedly prolongs disease-free survival when it is given as primary or adjuvant therapy in addition to surgery, chemo-therapy, and radiation to women with Her2/neu-positive breast cancers.

Erbitux (cetuximab) is another monoclonal antibody directed against the cancer cell surface portion of an EGFR tyrosine kinase protein that is a molecular cousin of Her2/neu. It has a checkered background because it was the cause of the ImClone insider stock manipulation scandal that involved Martha Stewart, but it has shown limited promise in some patients with colon cancer and may be promising in lung cancers that overexpress the normal receptor and do not respond to another smart drug called Iressa (to be discussed in more detail).

Other monoclonal antibodies have been armed with highly radioactive isotopes. The antibodies are unwittingly ingested by the cancer cells for which they have been designed, and the cancer cells are killed by the radiation. This is the radiation chemists' version of the Trojan horse and has been championed among others by the Fred Hutchinson Cancer Center in Seattle and by Memorial Sloan–Kettering Cancer Center in New York.

Though monoclonal antibodies have proven useful and may be very effective weapons in the attack on activated growth-promoting proteins that are the products of overexpressed oncogenes, the future depends on small molecules like Gleevec. These are the true smart drugs that can be taken by mouth, are much less expensive to manufacture, and are easily dose adjusted. Their downside is the development of drug resistance, but steps are being taken to deal with that menace, and new smart drugs are already in the clinical pipeline.

In June 2006, GlaxoSmithKline announced the results of preliminary trials of lapatinib or Tykerb, an orally active drug that hits Her2/neu in breast cancer. It is too early to know whether Tykerb will replace Herceptin, but the announcement illustrates the pace of discovery.

Iressa (gefitinib) and Tarceva (erlotinib) are two other newly developed smart drugs—small molecules that were designed to inhibit a particular EGFR tyrosine kinase protein that is present in patients with lung cancer. The history of those drugs is a cautionary tale.

Astra Zeneca is a large international pharmaceutical company with headquarters in Britain. The company's laboratories worked for years to develop Iressa as an inhibitor of one of the EGFR tyrosine kinases. The receptor interacts with a growth factor known as EGF, and when it does, it tells the cancer cell to divide. The company had reason to believe that many lung cancers contain a superabundance of EGFR protein and would therefore be likely to die when confronted by an EGFR inhibitor. To that end, the company produced the small molecule called Iressa. At about the same time, Genentech, a biotech/pharmaceutical company in California, produced Tarceva, a very similar drug. In 2002, Astra Zeneca started a clinical trial involving nearly seventeen hundred lung cancer patients, half of whom received Iressa. In 2003, the FDA approved the drug for the last-ditch treatment of lung cancer.

In 2004, startling reports were published by Bill Sellers, Bruce Johnson, Pasi Jänne, and Matt Meyerson at Dana-Farber Cancer Institute, together with Japanese investigators, who had been collecting and analyzing samples of lung cancer cells from patients at Dana-Farber, the Brigham and Women's Hospital, and from Japan, and by Tom Lynch and Dan Haber and their colleagues at Massachusetts General Hospital. Both groups came up with the same surprising findings. A small percentage of lung cancers (perhaps as few as 5 or 10 percent) of nonsmoking American patients and a larger percentage of Japanese patients, particularly Japanese women, have mutations in one copy of the gene for an EGFR tyrosine kinase. The mutation leads to the production of a fearsomely active oncoprotein that floods the cancer cell with signals that encourage cell division and prevent cell death. Just as Gleevec binds to the ATP-binding pocket of kit, Iressa jumps into the ATP-binding pocket of the EGFR oncoprotein and renders it inoperable by preventing ATP from getting into its bed in the protein. Devoid of ATP, the oncoprotein stops signaling. The cancer cells, deprived of their message to divide and their invitation to immortality, can only die.

The discovery strongly suggested that Iressa would only work effectively in the approximately 10 percent of lung cancer patients who have mutated EGFR genes that produce a hyperactive EGFR protein, just as mutated abl genes produce a hyperactive abl protein in CML and mutated kit produces GIST. The Iressa-sensitive mutated EGFR holds ATP in its pocket continuously and thereby signals lung cancer cells to divide whether they see EGF or not. The drug blocks access of ATP to its pocket and quickly kills lung cancer cells if they bear the mutated hyperactive receptor. However, the 90 percent of lung cancer patients who have the usual or increased levels of normal EGFR protein gain little benefit from the treatment.

Late in 2004, Astra Zeneca was forced to announce that its large and expensive clinical trial was statistically negative. The company could not observe a clearly measurable effect of the drug on survival of the overall group that had received it (as compared to the control group). Had the company realized from the beginning that only a small subset of lung cancer patients would respond favorably, it would have set its sights and budgets accordingly. Unwittingly and certainly unwillingly, Astra Zeneca had produced a drug that effectively treats rare patients with mutant EGFR-bearing cancer cells whether they are lung cancers or perhaps cancers that arise in other organs.

Instead of well-earned pride and joy, the *New York Times* reported in 2005 that the company was being faced with the possibility that the FDA would order the drug to be taken off the U.S. market because it lacked efficacy in a large clinical trial in which patients who might benefit were a tiny minority. Such a draconian decision would be manifestly unwise. The point of the story is that oncologists must choose drugs that can help their patients. A minority of lung cancer patients do gain benefit from Iressa and Tarceva.

Iressa and Tarceva are not the only new smart drugs in clinical trials directed against tyrosine kinases. At the end of 2004, the prestigious journal *Nature Reviews: Cancer* devoted an entire issue to accounts of the many efforts of academic and pharmaceutical company researchers to define pathways such as kinases that cause cancer and to develop drugs to inhibit them. At least a score of well-defined gene mutations have already been found to produce oncoproteins that cause several different kinds of cancer. New methods of scanning of the entire genome of cancers utilizing assays such as SNP (single-nucleotide polymorphism) and CGH (comparative genomic hybridization) array promise to reveal the genetic bases of cancers with great precision.

Many of the mutations will not be important, but each cancer is likely to have one to five critical mutations that drive the tumor. We need many more drugs that deal with those critical mutations—the oncoproteins that they induce or the deletions of key sniffing proteins that they generate. It is encouraging that so many have already appeared. Even the cynical *Wall Street Journal* editorialized on February 23, 2006, that cancer mortality has begun to decline and "new drug therapies, less punishing and invasive than surgery or chemotherapy, have been developed." The editors cannot help adding "thanks to the incentives of a private medical marketplace."

Flt3, for example, is the receptor tyrosine kinase that Scott Armstrong found to be abnormal in Mario's MLL leukemia and in other forms of childhood leukemia. Gary Gilliland and James Griffin at Dana-Farber and the Brigham and Women's Hospital have found flt3 mutations in adult leukemias. That gene can misbehave in two ways: a normal flt3 gene can be overexpressed like Her2/neu in breast cancer and different members of the EGFR family in colon cancer and lung cancer, or it can be mutated to a hyperactive state like abl in CML, kit in GIST, and EGFR in 5 to 10 percent of lung cancers. Several pharmaceutical companies have made drugs (currently identified with numbers instead of names) that inhibit hyperactive flt3. The clinical trials to evaluate those drugs are now in progress in several cancer centers. The early results are promising, but resistance will still be an issue.

Velcade (bortezomib) is another smart drug of a totally different class. It has nothing to do with tyrosine kinases as far as we know. It is a perfect example of the value of casting a broad net to search for useful and relatively nontoxic anticancer compounds. Just as intact humans accumulate rubbish, so do their individual cells, and cancer cells are no exception. Proteins, fats, and complex carbohydrates break down in cells and must be disposed of. The cell neatly degrades waste proteins using specialized destroyers called proteosomes.

Velcade inhibits proteosome formation, allowing proteins to accumulate inappropriately in the cell. Remarkably, Velcade can kill multiple myeloma, a malignancy of bone marrow–derived antibody-producing cells that individually produce a great deal of protein. Much of it accumulates in cells as junk and is disposed of in proteosomes. Velcade stops the disposal process. Current trials suggest that the drug leads to therapeutic responses in 30 percent of patients with multiple myeloma. Its mode of action is not entirely clear, but it unleashes the death pathway in myeloma cells. And Velcade, in combination with Adriamycin, a carpet-bombing drug, has powerful activity in a range of cancers.

A line of approach to smart drug development that has received a great deal of public attention in the past several years has focused on the supporting structure of tumors rather than the cancer cells themselves. As my colleagues Doug Hanahan at the University of California in San

Francisco and Bob Weinberg at the Massachusetts Institute of Technology have emphasized, tumors are like organs that reside within organs. A breast cancer grows initially as a mini-organ within breast tissue. To grow, it must develop a supporting structure complete with fibrous tissue, immune cells, and blood vessels. Recent experiments carried out in mice that are made genetically deficient in their ability to produce blood vessels clearly demonstrate that such mice are almost incapable of harboring tumors. (They have many other defects in blood vessel physiology as well.)

In 1972, Judah Folkman, a brilliant pediatric surgeon at Children's Hospital in Boston, conceived of the idea of attacking the established blood vessel support of cancers in order to starve the entire tumor and hence kill the cancer cells. He called the approach antiangiogenesis. His ideas and his results in mouse tumor models galvanized the news media after James Watson, one of the founders of the DNA revolution in biology, unguardedly advised an alert reporter that Folkman's approach to antiangiogenic therapy would soon become a cancer cure. Thus far, there have been bits of evidence that an attack on human tumor blood vessels may be an effective approach to human cancers, especially those that are particularly dependent on the angiogenesis process.

One monoclonal antibody called Avastin or bevacizumab binds to vascular endothelial growth factor (VEGF) and removes it from the circulation. VEGF normally combines with a family of receptor tyrosine kinases collectively called VEGFR, the latter expressed largely but not exclusively in the endothelial cells that line the blood vessels. Complicating any analysis of manipulation of VEGFR is the fact that the family of receptors can be detected in a wide variety of normal and malignant cells. In addition to the endothelial cells that line the blood vessels, the receptor family is found on bone marrow stem cells, pancreatic duct cells, retinal cells, testicular cells, and on cancer cells of the kidney, bladder, ovaries, and brain. Therefore, any results of treatment directed against tumor blood vessels must be analyzed very carefully to be sure that the targeted receptors are not also present on the cancer cells themselves.

Clinical trials suggest that antiangiogenic treatment may be effective in tumors that are particularly reliant on the angiogenesis pathway. Kidney cancer is one example. One of the fundamental molecular lesions in the DNA of kidney cancer tumors causes the angiogenesis pathway to become activated, resulting in tumors that are extraordinarily rich in blood vessels. The orally active raf inhibitor sorafanib has recently been approved for kidney cancer, in which it has significant activity, probably because a secondary target of the drug is the VEGF receptor on blood vessel cells. In addition, Avastin, the antibody that binds and eliminates VEGF, has led to small improvements in the survival of patients with colon cancer and lung cancer, but only when given with carpet-bombing chemotherapy.

Though Avastin is not a breakthrough drug and more recent studies have strongly suggested that the antibody may damage the normal blood vessels of the heart, any reproducible effect of the antibody may provide proof that an attack on tumor blood vessels can represent a smart approach to cancer treatment. If the principle is correct, the system can be improved. In fact, Regeneron, a small biotech company, has created a molecule that it claims literally traps all the VEGF in the blood and prevents it from reacting with its receptors. The trapping molecule has a tremendous effect on mouse tumors. Whether this approach will be of any value in humans with cancer remains to be seen, but the results prove that better inhibitors of tumor blood vessel growth may be very useful. Toward that end, scientists at the Massachusetts Institute of Technology have devised a special compound that releases both antiangiogenic and chemotherapeutic drugs simultaneously in an experimental tumor in mice. The results are somewhat promising, but translation of their finding to an effective treatment for humans may be difficult.

Many drugs are currently touted as antiangiogenic agents, but they may have other effects that explain their activities. The fascinating work goes on. If tumor control could be achieved by inhibition of the blood vessels that nourish the tumors, a single smart drug could be enormously effective in a very broad array of cancers. Since the endothelial cells that line the blood vessels have stable genes, the development of resistance to antiangiogenics would be far less frequent in those cells than is the case for genetically unstable cancer cells.

Not discussed here in any detail but certainly worthy of mention is another very promising area of cancer treatment: the production of cancer vaccines. One type of vaccine is designed to boost the immune response of a patient against his or her own cancer cells. The theory is based on the clear fact that the surface of cancer cells is not normal, and therefore cancer cells should be successfully attacked and destroyed by the immune system. Unfortunately, cancer cells have developed several protective ways to avoid such an attack, but the work is in full swing and those who pursue it remain encouraged for good reason.

A second and clearly effective cancer vaccination approach is one that prevents cancer. Cervical cancer, for example, is caused by a papilloma virus that is spread by sexual intercourse. Merck has developed an effective vaccine against that virus. Incredibly, the FDA, now in the toils of the George W. Bush administration, delayed approval of that excellent product because religious right partisans do not want to approve any product that might enhance sexual freedom. No one should be surprised. Science policy in the Bush administration can only be described as absurd and dangerous. That some of our best scientific agencies survive is a tribute to a few remarkable government officers. Fortunately, an external FDA advisory group favorably reviewed the vaccine data during the spring of 2006. Hence the reluctant and politically controlled leadership of the FDA was forced to approve the vaccine.

We have every reason to assume that the new approaches to precise molecular detection of the defective genes that cause cancer will be very likely to provide important new targets for smart-drug therapy. But we must also assume that cancer cells will figure out a way to continue to mutate in order to salvage the pathways that they require for their survival. Thus, second- and third-generation smart drugs will have to be made until the targeted cancer cells run out of mutation options and finally succumb for good.

Such an effort represents a formidable economic challenge to pharmaceutical companies. Each drug requires millions of dollars in development costs, and each product might well be sold to an ever-smaller group of patients because patients' cancers may have quite unique molecular signatures. In our pharmaceutical company culture, private companies must be financially independent and responsible to their stockholders. They cannot be expected to manufacture highly expensive drugs without assurance that they will be paid for their investment and earn a profit. They assume that they must make drugs that will be prescribed to hundreds of thousands of patients—not a few hundred.

There is, of course, plenty of waste in drug company budgets, particularly in marketing, but the costs that must be envisaged to prepare second-, third-, and fourth-generation smart drugs go well beyond any marketing savings that drug companies may be able to achieve. Given the understandable hostility to drug prices that permeates our society and the anger that is generated when pharmaceutical companies ruthlessly establish prices based on what the market will bear, it may be difficult to conceive of a helping hand to pharmaceutical companies. But some sort of public/private partnership involving the National Cancer Institute, the academic medical centers, and the pharmaceutical companies may be required if the flow of new smart drugs is to reach the maximum permitted by scientific knowledge.

Cost resistance is already with us. An arm of the National Health Service of the United Kingdom has recently denied Herceptin as adjuvant therapy for a thirty-six-year-old woman with Her2/neu-positive breast cancer. The case made international news in 2006. Avastin and Erbitux are already well beyond the reach of most patients on the basis of cost.

There is one saving grace on the horizon. One of the huge expenses of drug development is the clinical trial. In order to determine whether a drug is effective, large numbers of patients must be treated and their cancers measured during the course of treatment. Many of these expensive trials are negative or marginal, and they cost a king's ransom. Fortunately, a much better analytical tool is on the horizon.

Physicists and engineers are rapidly developing imaging instruments such as positron emission tomography (PET) scanners and magnetic resonance imaging (MRI) machines that can visualize an astonishingly small number of cancer cells and determine whether they are dead or alive. With the use of those instruments and new testing compounds, it would be possible to determine very quickly whether a new drug kills cancer cells. Replacement of laborious, expensive, and lengthy clinical trials with rapid imaging would save a fortune and decrease disability by avoiding exposure of patients to worthless drugs. The further development of imaging systems will require a substantial but worthwhile investment by cancer centers. Modern imaging science is the wave of the future in therapeutic cancer research.

The bottom line is that smart drugs for cancer have already been developed. We simply need a lot more of them, and we need to do the brute force laboratory work required to establish the molecular signatures of every invasive cancer that extends beyond the range of surgery and afflicts thousands each year. With the diagnostic data in hand, we will match molecular signature with correctly chosen smart drug combinations and kill cancer. Recent work by Todd Golub and Scott Armstrong and their colleagues shows that the approach is sound.

Despite recent progress, efforts will not be easy. There will be technical pitfalls in the analytic laboratories, difficulties in obtaining sufficient samples of pure cancer cells for analysis, and obstacles in development of procedures. And even when all of the technical problems involved in searching the genome for mutations that convert normal genes to oncogenes are solved, there will be further hurdles to overcome. It is increasingly clear that simple travel up and down the genome of cancer cells looking for mutations, amplifications, or deletions of genes responsible for cancer is a start but not an entire solution.

Cancer is a disorder of cell growth regulation. Growth and differentiation of cells is certainly affected by gene mutations, but some genes may be perfectly normal and still be dysregulated. They may be dysregulated to the point of oncogenicity by other proteins in the cell, the genes for which are very distant from the gene that influences cancer cell growth. For example, some patients with Ken's type of GIST might have perfectly normal kit genes in the tumor cells, but the output of the tumor-causing kit genes might be greatly amplified by a protein that has in turn been mutated. Laborious sequencing of the kit genes in the tumor would be unrewarding, but kit would still be the villain. We call such tumors epigenetic cancers, and we are beginning to learn that epigenetics may play a very important role in the pathogenesis of many cancers. So "simple" gene analysis is a very necessary first start toward identifying gene targets for smart drugs. But we will have to develop the epigenetic targets as well.

Furthermore, we must accept the fact that cancer cells remain incredibly evasive because of their ability to mutate further in the face of an onslaught and because the cells in a cancer may be heterogeneous. While most are clones of one another, a few so-called cancer stem cells may be driven by entirely different genes, none of which are affected by a particular group of drugs. In many cases, we will not wipe out the cancer but only keep it at bay. In effect, we will manage some cases as chronic diseases, keeping the cancer suppressed as we vary the combinations of drugs and monitor the patients with increasingly sensitive imaging methods. But we will keep our patients with us much longer, and we will do it with far less toxicity.

It will not be easy. But if a collaborative effort among oncologists; basic, population, information, and imaging scientists; pharmaceutical companies; private foundations; and government is successfully established, we will see the positive effects of the new therapies on cancer mortality in the next twenty years. The pressure applied by the families and friends of Mario, Joan, and Ken, and the thousands who share their plight, will eventually direct us toward success. To paraphrase Winston Churchill: "We are not at the beginning of the end, but we are at the end of the beginning." The cancer treatment revolution engendered by smart drugs is on the way, and the sooner the better. We owe this revolution to the memory of Ken and to the thousands of patients like him who have succumbed or depend on us right now for a better future.

# Glossary

**4G10** A monoclonal antibody that detects phosphotyrosine and hence an activated tyrosine kinase.

**5-fluorouracil** An anticancer drug that inhibits DNA repair and synthesis and thereby reduces the growth of cancer cells.

**6-MP** *See* 6-mercaptopurine.

**6-mercaptopurine** An anticancer drug that inhibits DNA repair and synthesis, thus reducing the growth of cancer cells, particularly leukemic cells. It is also used as an immunosuppressive agent.

**Abelson virus** or **Abelson murine leukemia virus (Ab-MLV)** A retrovirus that triggers a type of leukemia in mice.

**abl** A normal mammalian gene that produces a tyrosine kinase enzyme that promotes growth.

**abscess** A localized collection of pus in any body part that results from invasion of bacteria. *Staphylococcus aureus* infection is a common cause.

**ACTH** Adrenocorticotropic hormone; a hormone secreted by the pituitary gland that controls the development and functioning of the adrenal cortex, including its secretion of steroids, glucocorticoids, and androgens.

**Actinomycin D** *See* dactinomycin.

**acute lymphoblastic leukemia (ALL)** A hematological malignancy marked by the unchecked multiplication of immature lymphoid cells in the bone marrow, blood, and body tissues.

**acute myeloblastic leukemia (AML)** A group of hematological malignancies in which neoplastic cells develop from myeloid (germ eaters), monocytic (debris eaters), erythrocytic (red cell), or megakaryocytic (platelet) precursors.

**adenosine triphosphate (ATP)** Present in all cells, it is formed when energy is released from food during cell metabolism. Cells contain enzymes such as tyrosine kinases that split ATP into ADP, phosphate, and energy, which is then available for cellular functions such as mitosis (cell division).

**adjuvant chemotherapy** The giving of drugs to eradicate malignant cells that may remain in the body after surgery or radiation therapy.

**adrenalectomy** Excision of one or both adrenal glands.

**Adriamycin** An anthracycline-based anticancer drug that inhibits DNA repair and synthesis, thus reducing the growth of cancer cells. Generic name: doxorubicin.

**AIDS** Acquired immunodeficiency syndrome, a late stage of infection in human immunodeficiency virus (HIV).

**albumin** One of a group of proteins widely distributed in plant and animal tissues. In the blood, albumin helps to maintain blood volume and blood pressure.

**ALL**  *See* acute lymphoblastic leukemia.

**amethopterin**  *See* methotrexate.

**amino acid**  Any of a class of nitrogenous organic compounds that are essential components of proteins. They are the building blocks of proteins and the end products of protein digestion.

**aminopterin**  A folic acid antagonist that binds and inactivates dihydrofolate reductase and thereby inhibits folic acid metabolism. Used to treat acute leukemia.

**AML**  *See* acute myeloblastic leukemia.

**AML1**  Acute myeloid leukemia 1 gene. Often involved in translocations associated with leukemia.

**AMN107**  *See* nilotinib.

**analogue**  A compound that is structurally similar to another.

**androgen**  Substance such as testosterone or androsterone that stimulates the development of male characteristics.

**anemia**  A deficiency in red blood cells, in hemoglobin, or in volume of blood.

**anthracyclines**  A class of anticancer drugs that inhibit DNA repair and synthesis, thus reducing the growth of cancer cells. They are used in the treatment of solid organ cancers and leukemias.

**antiangiogenic therapy**  The blocking of the formation of new blood vessels, especially the blood vessels that grow under the influence of malignant tumors.

**antibiotic**  A natural or synthetic substance that destroys microorganisms or inhibits their growth.

**antibody**  A protein produced by B-lymphocytes in response to a unique antigen. Each antibody molecule combines with a specific antigen. The binding of an antigen on the surface of an infecting organism by an antibody encourages the ingestion and killing of the organism by granulocytes or macrophages. All antibodies, except natural antibodies (e.g., antibodies to different blood types), are made by B-cells stimulated by a nonself antigen, typically a foreign protein, polysaccharide (a complex sugar molecule), or nucleic acid (the constituents of DNA and RNA). Antibodies against self antigens are called autoantibodies and often cause disease.

**anticoagulant**  An agent that prevents or delays blood coagulation. Common anticoagulants include heparin, sodium citrate, and warfarin (Coumadin).

**antiemetic drug**  An agent that prevents or relieves nausea and vomiting.

**antigen**  A substance that induces the B-lymphocytes of the immune system to produce antibodies against it.

**antimetabolite**  A class of antineoplastic drugs used to treat cancer. Antimetabolites are structurally similar to vitamins, coenzymes, or other substances essential for growth and division of normal and neoplastic cells. These drugs are most effective against rapidly growing tumors.

**antioncogene**  A gene that produces a protein that suppresses the growth of cells. Its absence in a cell may lead to cancer. *See* tumor suppressor gene.

**arabinoside**  Gum sugar, a pentose (5-carbon sugar).

**AraC**  Cytarabine (or cytosine arabinoside), an antineoplastic drug of the antimetabolite class.

**aromatase inhibitors**  Drugs that block aromatase, an enzyme essential for the synthesis of estrogen from androgen. A number of these agents have been developed to treat breast cancer, which is often an estrogen-responsive malignancy.

**asparaginase** An enzyme derived from the bacterium *Escherichia coli*. The enzyme destroys the amino acid asparagine, thus inhibiting protein synthesis in and growth of ALL cells.

**asparagine** Aminosuccinic acid, an amino acid.

**Aspergillus** A genus of fungi comprising more than six hundred species of molds. Highly invasive in immunocompromised patients such as those receiving combination chemotherapy for cancer.

**aspirate** To draw in or out by suction.

**assays** The analysis of a substance to determine its constituents and the relative proportion of each.

**ATP** *See* adenosine triphosphate.

**Avastin** Drug that inhibits the action of a receptor tyrosine kinase called VEGFR, one function of which is the formation of new blood vessels that cancer cells require for growth. Generic name: bevacizumab.

**axilla** The armpit.

**azacytidine** A rarely used anticancer drug that is incorporated into DNA and blocks its proper function, thereby inhibiting DNA repair and synthesis and reducing cancer cell growth.

**basal cell carcinoma** A malignancy typically found on skin exposed to sun or other forms of ultraviolet light.

**Bay 43-9006** *See* sorafenib.

**BCC** *See* basal cell carcinoma.

**bcr** *See* breakpoint cluster region.

**bcr-abl** Oncogene and oncoprotein responsible for Philadelphia chromosome–positive chronic myelogenous (myelocytic) leukemia.

**benign** Not recurrent or progressive; nonmalignant.

**bevacizumab** *See* Avastin.

**biopsy** The obtaining of a representative tissue sample for microscopic examination, usually to establish a diagnosis.

**blockade** Inhibition (usually by a drug) of a cellular pathway that controls a cellular function.

**blood** The fluid that circulates through the heart, arteries, veins, and capillaries, carrying nourishment and oxygen to the tissues and taking away waste matter and carbon dioxide. It also carries granulocytes and monocytes (germ-eating cells), lymphocytes that influence immunity, and platelets (the initiators of clotting).

**B-lymphocyte** A cell formed from pluripotent stem cells in the bone marrow. It migrates to the spleen, lymph nodes, and other peripheral lymphoid tissue, where it comes in contact with foreign antigens and becomes a mature antibody-producing plasma cell.

**BMS-354825** *See* desatinib.

**BMT** *See* bone marrow transplantation.

**bone marrow** The soft tissue that fills the cavities of the bones and in which blood cell production occurs after fetal life.

**bone marrow transplantation (BMT)** Transfer of bone marrow from one individual to another; a procedure in which a large needle with a syringe attached is inserted into the pelvic bone of a donor, and about a pint of marrow and blood cells containing blood stem cells is sucked out. The cells are then given by vein to a compatible recipient. The donor stem cells establish blood cell production in the recipient.

**BRCA1** and **BRCA2** Genes that produce proteins involved in DNA repair. Their absence greatly increases the risk of breast and ovarian cancer. Therefore, inactivating mutations of these genes indicate a likelihood of breast cancer and ovarian cancer.

**breakpoint cluster region (bcr)** DNA on chromosome 22 that is the site of fractures on that chromosome that accept a fragment of chromosome 9, which contains the abl gene. This translocation creates bcr/abl. The modified chromosome 22 is known as the Philadelphia chromosome and is diagnostic of chronic myelogenous leukemia.

**breast cancer** A malignant neoplasm (usually an adenocarcinoma) of the breast.

**breast lobe** *See* lobe of breast.

**bromodeoxyuridine** An antimetabolite that is incorporated into DNA, where it inhibits repair and DNA synthesis, thereby reducing the growth of cancer cells.

**CA** Cytoxan (cyclophosphamide) and anthracyclines. A combination of anticancer drugs used in the management of breast cancer.

**c-abl** The normal abl gene, a proto-oncogene.

**Cajal cell tumor** *See* gastrointestinal stromal tumor.

**cancer** Malignant neoplasia marked by the uncontrolled growth of cells, often with invasion of healthy tissues locally or throughout the body.

**cancer genetics** The study of cancer genes.

**capecitabine** An antimetabolite that is converted in the body to 5-fluorouracil. The latter is incorporated into DNA, where it inhibits DNA repair and synthesis, thus reducing the growth of cancer cells. It is particularly used in breast cancer. Trade name: Xeloda.

**carcinoma** A new growth or malignant tumor that occurs in epithelial tissue and may infiltrate local tissues or produce metastases.

**CAT scan** *See* computer-assisted tomography.

**cell** A mass of protoplasm containing a nucleus or nuclear material; the structural unit of all animals and plants. A typical cell has a nucleus surrounded by cytoplasm.

**cell separation** The separation of cells from one another based on physical or chemical properties. Cell separation techniques are used to collect uniform populations of cells from tissues or fluids in which many different cell types are present.

**central nervous system prophylaxis** Preventive measures to kill cancer cells lurking in the brain and spinal cord where they may not be reached by oral or intravenous chemotherapy.

**cervical cancer** A malignant neoplasm of the cervix of the uterus caused by the human papilloma virus.

**CGH** *See* comparative genomic hybridization.

**chemo-radiation therapy** Drug and radiation therapy.

**chemoradiosensitive** Responds to both chemotherapy and radiation therapy.

**chemotherapy** Treatment of disease by antibiotics or anticancer drugs.

**Chloromycetin** An antibacterial drug. Generic name: chloramphenicol.

**CHOP** Cyclophosphamide, Adriamycin (hydroxydaunomycin), vincristine (Oncovin), and prednisone; a combination chemotherapy regimen for non-Hodgkin's lymphoma.

**choriocarcinoma** An extremely rare, very malignant neoplasm that arises in the chorion, a membrane surrounding the fetus.

**choriongonadotropic hormone**  A hormone produced by the chorion and in large amounts by choriocarcinoma. It can be found in the urine and provides the basis of a pregnancy test as well as an approach to monitor choriocarcinoma therapy.

**chromosomal translocation**  The alteration of a chromosome by transfer of a portion of it either to another chromosome or to another portion of the same chromosome.

**chromosome**  A linear strand made of DNA and protein that carries genetic information. Genes are sequences of DNA that are largely contained within chromosomes. Normally present in the somatic (nongerm) cells of humans are forty-six chromosomes, including two sex-determining chromosomes (either X and Y in males or X and X in females). There are twenty-three chromosomes in the germ cells—an X in ova and either an X or a Y in sperm.

**chronic myelogenous leukemia (CML)**  A hematological malignancy marked by a sustained increase in the number of granulocytes, splenic enlargement, and a specific cytogenetic anomaly—the Philadelphia chromosome—in the bone marrow and blood of more than 90 percent of patients.

**cisplatin**  An anticancer drug that contains platinum.

**clinical imaging**  The production of a picture, image, or shadow that represents the object being investigated. In diagnostic medicine, the classic technique for imaging is radiographic or X-ray examination. The more modern methods (CT, MRI, and PET) are particularly applicable in the diagnosis and treatment of cancer.

**clinical trial**  A carefully designed and executed investigation of the therapeutic and toxic effects of a drug administered to human subjects.

**CMF**  Combination chemotherapy with cyclophosphamide, methotrexate, and 5-fluorouracil.

**CML**  *See* chronic myelogenous leukemia.

**colitis**  Inflammation of the colon.

**colon**  The large intestine from the end of the ileum to the anal canal that surrounds the anus; divided into the ascending, transverse, descending, and sigmoid or pelvic colon.

**colonoscopy**  Visualization of the lower gastrointestinal tract; most often refers to insertion of a flexible endoscope through the anus to inspect the entire colon.

**combination chemotherapy**  The use of two or more anticancer drugs.

**comparative genomic hybridization (CGH)**  A method to analyze loss or gain of genes in tumor cells.

**computer-assisted tomography (CAT or CT scan)**  Computerized axial tomography scan. *See* computerized tomography.

**computerized tomography (CT)**  A radiographic technique that selects a level in the body and blurs out structures above and below that plane, leaving a clear image of the selected anatomy.

**core biopsy**  Removal of a tissue sample with a hollow needle. The tissue is then evaluated under a microscope.

**cortisone**  A hormone isolated from the cortex of the adrenal gland and also prepared synthetically. It regulates the metabolism of fats, carbohydrates, sodium, potassium, and proteins, and is also used as an anti-inflammatory agent.

**CT**  *See* computerized tomography.

**cyclophosphamide**  An antineoplastic drug that chemically cross-links DNA. It has also been used as an immunosuppressive agent in organ transplantation. Trade name: Cytoxan.

**cyst**  A closed sac or pouch with a definite wall that contains fluid, semifluid, or solid material.

**cytarabine**  Also known as AraC and cytosine arabinoside. A drug originally developed as an antileukemic agent, but it is also used in treating *Herpesvirus hominis* infections that cause either keratitis or encephalitis.

**cytogenetics**  The study of the structure and function of chromosomes.

**cytosine**  A pyrimidine base that is part of DNA and RNA. In DNA it is paired with guanine.

**cytosine arabinoside**  *See* cytarabine.

**Cytoxan**  *See* cyclophosphamide.

**dactinomycin**  An anticancer drug of the antibiotic class that prevents cancer cells from dividing. Trade name: Actinomycin D.

**dasatinib**  An anticancer drug that inhibits certain tyrosine kinses. Initially tested in patients with chronic myelogenous leukemia (CML).

**daunomycin**  An anticancer drug in the anthracycline class.

**DCIS**  *See* ductal carcinoma in situ.

**deoxyribonucleic acid (DNA)**  A molecule that carries genetic information for all organisms except the RNA viruses. DNA consists of adenine, guanine, cytosine, thymine, deoxyribose, and phosphate.

**dermatitis**  A rash marked by itching, redness, and swelling.

**DHFR**  Dihydrofolate reductase. An enzyme central to the metabolism of folic acid.

**dissection**  The separation and delineation of tissues for study.

**DNA**  *See* deoxyribonucleic acid.

**dominant**  In genetics, concerning a trait or characteristic that is expressed in the offspring, although it is carried on only one of the homologous pair of chromosomes.

**drug infusion**  The injection of liquid drugs into a vein for therapeutic purposes.

**ductal carcinoma in situ (DCIS)**  A cluster of malignant cells in the mammary ducts.

**EGFR**  *See* epidermal growth factor receptor.

**embolism**  The sudden obstruction of a blood vessel by debris such as blood clots, plaque, masses of bacteria, or cancer cells, all of which may lodge in the blood vessels and obstruct the circulation.

**enzyme**  A protein capable of accelerating the chemical reaction of a substance (the substrate) without being destroyed or altered. Enzymes are reaction specific in that they act only on certain substrates.

**epidemic**  An outbreak of a disease that affects a large group of people in a geographic region or defined population.

**epidermal growth factor receptor (EGFR)**  A receptor tyrosine kinase found on the surface of cells to which epidermal growth factor (EGF) binds. When EGF attaches to EGFR, it activates the tyrosine kinase component of EGFR, triggering reactions that cause the cells to grow and multiply. EGFR relays instructions to cells to grow and divide and to ignore signals telling them to die.

**epigenetic cancers**  Cancer induced by nongene molecules that bind to normal genes and change their expression into RNA and protein.

**epithelial cancer** Cancer derived from epithelial cells, such as breast, colon, and many lung cancers.

**epithelial cells** One of the cells forming the epithelial surfaces of membranes, ducts, and skin.

**ER** *See* estrogen receptor.

**Erbitux** An anticancer drug that targets one of the class of epidermal growth factor receptors. Generic name: cetuximab.

**ERK** Extracellular signal-regulated kinase. A signaling molecule that is part of the RAS signaling pathway.

**erlotinib** *See* Tarceva.

**erythromycin** An antibiotic used primarily to treat gram-positive and atypical microorganisms such as streptococci, mycoplasma, and legionella.

**estrogen** Any natural or artificial substance that induces estrus and the development of female sex characteristics.

**estrogen receptor (ER)** The receptor protein in the cell to which estrogen binds. Breast cancers that express estrogen receptors are more responsive to estrogen-blocking drugs such as tamoxifen than tumors that lack these receptors.

**estrogen receptor–positive breast cancer** Breast tumors with estrogen receptors present.

**ET-743 (ecteinascidin 743)** A marine anticancer drug found in the tissues of sea squirts. Trade names: Trabectedin, Yondelin.

**exchange transfusion** The removal of one patient's blood and its replacement with blood donated by others.

**FACS** *See* fluorescence-activated cell sorting.

**Faslodex** An inhibitor of estrogen receptor used in the hormone therapy of estrogen-dependent breast cancer. Generic name: fulvestrant. *See also* tamoxifen.

**fibrocystic** Consisting of fibrous tissue and cysts.

**fibrotic strands** A single thread of fiber of fibrous tissue.

**fine-needle biopsy** The removal of tissue through a narrow-gauge needle.

**flt3** A receptor tyrosine kinase, a signaling enzyme involved in cellular growth regulation.

**flt3 inhibitor** A drug that inhibits the activity of flt3 and thereby reduces the growth of certain leukemic cells that depend on the enzyme. Certain mutations of the flt3 gene may lead to hyperactive flt3 enzyme and continuous growth signaling. The inhibitor can block that hyperactivity, thus killing the leukemic cells.

**fluorescence-activated cell sorting (FACS)** A method of separating cells by selectively tagging them with colored fluorescent dyes bound to specific cellular structures or molecules.

**folic acid** A water-soluble B-complex vitamin needed for DNA synthesis; occurring naturally in green leafy vegetables, beans, and yeast.

**fungi** Organisms that grow as single cells, as in yeast, or as multicellular filamentous colonies, as in molds and mushrooms. Some fungi are highly infectious, particularly in immunodeficient patients such as those with AIDS and those who undergo aggressive cancer chemotherapy.

**gastrointestinal stromal tumor (GIST)** Uncommon tumor of the GI tract that arises in cells found in the wall of the GI tract; called the interstitial cells of Cajal (ICCs).

**gene** A sequence of base pairs in the DNA molecule that encodes the synthesis of one particular messenger RNA and protein molecule. Genes are the basic units of heredity. Hereditary traits are most often controlled by pairs of genes in the same position on a pair of chromosomes. If a mutation on only one gene of a pair causes a functional change in a protein, it is called a dominant gene. If both members of a pair must be mutated to produce a change, the gene is called recessive. The X chromosome is paired only in females. Hence males may carry defects due to a gene mutation on one X chromosome.

**gene amplification** Excessive replication of DNA to form multiple copies of a specific gene or genes.

**gene expression** The process by which genetic information is converted into messenger RNA molecules and then into proteins.

**gene regulation** Control of gene expression.

**genetics** The study of heredity and its variations and the study of the genome.

**genome** The complete set of genes on chromosomes and thus the entire genetic information present in a cell.

**GIST** *See* gastrointestinal stromal tumor.

**Gleevec** or **Glivec** *See* imatinib.

**glucose** A simple sugar that is the end product of carbohydrate digestion. Within cells, glucose is used to synthesize the pentose sugars, ribose and deoxyribose, for RNA and DNA.

**granulocyte** A leukocyte that ingests bacteria and kills the germ with proteins in the granules of its cytoplasm and with toxic oxygen species.

**hematoma** A swelling, usually comprised of clotted blood, caused by a break in a blood vessel.

**heme** A nonprotein insoluble iron compound found in hemoglobin. It is responsible for the color and oxygen-carrying properties of hemoglobin. There is one heme bound to each of the four globin chains of hemoglobin. Heme is also a component of myoglobin, the oxygen-carrying protein in muscle.

**hemoglobin** The oxygen-carrying protein in red cells. It contains four heme groups and four chains of globin, which together can bind oxygen in the lungs and release it in the tissues.

**hemorrhage** Blood loss. The escape of blood from the vessels.

**hemorrhagic** Marked by hemorrhage or blood loss.

**Her2/neu** Also known as ErbB-2, it is a member of the epidermal growth factor receptor (EGFR) family, the members of which are receptor tyrosine kinases. Her2/neu is a cell membrane surface-bound tyrosine kinase involved in the signal transduction pathways leading to cell growth and differentiation. When the Her2/neu gene is amplified (as it is in about 25 percent of breast cancers), the cancers contain excessive Her2/neu protein molecules and concomitant increased Her2/neu tyrosine kinase activity. It is notable for its role in the pathogenesis of breast cancer and as a target of treatment.

**Herceptin** A monoclonal antibody against Her2/neu protein and therefore effective in women with Her2/neu–positive breast cancer. Generic name: trastuzumab.

**heterogeneous** Of unlike natures or composed of unlike substances.

**hin1** A gene with high expression in normal breast duct cells (high in normal) and low in breast cancer.

**Hodgkin's disease** A malignant lymphoma. Early disease (stage 1 or 2) is present in one or a few lymph nodes. Widespread disease is disseminated to both sides of the diaphragm (stage 3) or throughout the body (stage 4).

**Hodgkin's lymphoma** *See* Hodgkin's disease.

**hormone** A substance originating in an organ, gland, or body part that is carried in the blood to another body part, stimulating that part to increase or decrease functional activity or to increase or decrease secretion of another hormone.

**H-ras** The Harvey rat sarcoma gene first described in a rat tumor virus that produces a hyperactive enzyme called GTPase (guanosine triphosphatase). GTPases are a large family of enzymes that can bind and hydrolyze GTP, a molecular cousin of adenosine triphosphate (ATP). GTPases play an important role in many cell functions including cell division. The normal enzyme (N-ras) is a GTPase that generates high-energy phosphorus from GTP (guanosine triphosphate). N-ras is therefore a proto-oncogene that normally participates in the signaling networks that stimulate cell growth. The mutated H- or K-ras forms are oncogenes that drive continuous cell growth. Mutant ras forms are commonly found in cancers. They are excellent drug targets, but no good ras inhibitor has been developed to date.

**hybridization** The binding of a DNA strand by a complementary strand.

**hydroxydaunomycin** An anticancer drug in the anthracycline family that is effective in treating a wide range of tumors.

**hyperactive protein** A mutated protein that acts as an oncoprotein and induces uncontrolled cell growth.

**ibuprofen** A nonsteroidal anti-inflammatory drug with fever-reducing and pain-relieving properties. Trade names: Advil, Motrin, Nuprin.

**imatinib** An anticancer drug that inserts into the ATP-binding pockets of the tyrosine kinase domains of bcr/abl, mutant kit, and mutant PDGFR—all oncoproteins. The drug binding prevents ATP access to the enzyme and therefore blocks tyrosine kinase activity. Imatinib is used with great benefit in patients with chronic myelogenous leukemia and gastrointestinal stromal tumor (GIST). Trade names: Gleevec, Glivec.

**immunodeficiency** The decreased or compromised ability to respond to antigenic stimuli with an appropriate immune response as the result of one or more disorders in B-cell– or T-cell–mediated immunity or phagocytic cells.

**immunosuppressive drug** Drug treatment that impairs immune responses.

**IMR** *See* intensity modulated radiation.

**informed consent** A voluntary agreement made by a well-advised and mentally competent patient to undergo treatment as part of a research study. The patient is provided full disclosure of information regarding the material risks, benefits of the proposed treatment, alternatives, and consequences of no treatment.

**Institutional Review Board (IRB)** A medical oversight committee that governs or regulates medical investigations involving human subjects. The purpose of the board is to protect the rights and health of participants in clinical trials.

**intensity modulated radiation (IMR)** Advanced radiation therapy that uses computer-controlled X-ray to deliver precise radiation doses to a malignant tumor.

**interleukin** A type of cytokine-a protein that enables communication among leukocytes and other cells active in inflammation or a specific immune response, resulting in a maximized response to a microorganism or other foreign antigen.

**invasive breast cancer (IVC)** Cancer that breaks through normal breast ducts and invades surrounding areas. These cancers can spread to other parts of the body through the bloodstream and lymphatic system.

**IRB** *See* Institutional Review Board.

**Iressa** An anticancer drug that inserts into the ATP-binding pocket of the tyrosine kinase domain of the mutant EGFR found in some cases of lung cancer, inhibiting the kinase activity and stopping cell division. Generic name: gefitnib.

**irradiation** The diagnostic or therapeutic application of any form of radiation to a patient. When used for treatment, photons, electrons, neutrons, or other ionizing radiation attack target tissues and cross-link DNA. The result is inhibition of cell replication.

**kinase** An enzyme protein that catalyzes the transfer of high-energy phosphate from ATP to an acceptor or substrate such as a tyrosine molecule within the protein. If tyrosine is the substrate (acceptor), the enzyme is called a tyrosine kinase. If the tyrosine kinase is activated by another protein, it is called a receptor tyrosine kinase. Other amino acids such as serine and threonine and many other molecules may also act as substrates. Kinase activity is central to the signaling processes that regulate cell growth.

**kit** A receptor tyrosine kinase that regulates cell growth and differentiation through the cell-signaling network. Mutations of kit are responsible for most cases of GIST.

**lapatinib** An anticancer drug that targets Her2/neu and may delay the progress of Her2-positive breast cancer. It can enter the spinal fluid and is effective in treating breast cancer metastatic to the brain.

**leukemia** A progressive, malignant disease of the marrow, spleen, and lymph nodes characterized by uncontrolled proliferation of white blood cells at the expense of normal blood cells.

**leukocyte** A white blood cell.

**Li-Fraumeni syndrome** Inactivating mutations of the p53 gene are responsible for this disease. It is an inherited condition in which individuals develop multiple primary tumors, including breast cancer, soft-tissue sarcoma, and brain tumors.

**linear accelerator** Increasing the transfer rate of ionizing radiation to soft tissue.

**lining cell** Cells such as endothelial cells that line the channels of lymph nodes, spleen, and bone marrow and the inner layer of blood vessels.

**lobe of breast (mammary gland)** One of the fifteen to twenty divisions of the glandular tissue of the breast separated by connective tissue, each possessing a duct (lobar duct) opening via the nipple.

**lobular** Consisting of lobes.

**lumpectomy** Surgical removal of a breast tumor and only limited surrounding tissue.

**lymphedema** An abnormal accumulation of tissue fluid (potential lymph) that can be caused by either impairment of normal uptake of tissue fluid by the lymphatic vessels or the excessive production of tissue fluid caused by obstruction to blood flow.

**lymph node**  Small kidney-shaped organs of lymphoid tissue that lie at intervals along the lymphatic vessels.

**lymphoblast**  An immature cell that gives rise to a lymphocyte.

**lymphoblastic leukemia**  *See* acute lymphoblastic anemia.

**lymphocyte**  A white blood cell (lymphocyte) responsible for much of the body's immune protection. Formed in the lymph nodes, spleen, tonsils, and thymus, where they can maximize contact with foreign antigens, these cells make up about one-quarter of all leukocytes in the blood of normal adults.

**lymphoma**  A malignant neoplasm originating from lymphocytes. *See also* Hodgkin's disease.

**magnetic resonance imaging (MRI)**  Based on radio wave-induced nuclear magnetic resonance of atoms (usually hydrogen) in the body, this diagnostic technique produces remarkably precise computerized images of tissues and organs and even small groups of individual cells.

**malignant**  In cancer, growths that enlarge, resist treatment, and metastasize.

**mammogram**  An X-ray of the breast.

**mammography**  Radiographic imaging of the breast to screen for and detect cancer.

**mastectomy**  Surgical removal of the breast. A patient undergoes this procedure as treatment for or prophylaxis against breast cancer.

**mdm2**  A gene that regulates the production of mdm2, a protein that binds and eliminates p53, the main driver of cell death. High levels of mdm2 activity in cancer cells therefore contribute to cancer cell immortality. Nutlin, an experimental drug, binds mdm2 and prevents it from interacting with p53.

**megaloblast**  A large, nucleated, abnormal red blood cell precursor seen in vitamin B12 and folic acid deficiency.

**mek**  A protein involved in the growth and survival of cancer cells that operates along the ras pathway.

**melanoma**  A malignant tumor of darkly pigmented cells (melanocytes) that often arises in a brown or black mole. The tumor can spread aggressively throughout the body.

**melphalan**  An antineoplastic drug of the nitrogen mustard class; a cross-linker of DNA.

**MEN**  *See* multiple endocrine neoplasia.

**MEN1**  Multiple endocrine neoplasia type 1 gene. This gene has inactivating mutations in MEN. Therefore, it is a tumor suppressor gene.

**meningitis**  Inflammation of the membranes of the spinal cord or brain, usually but not always caused by an infectious illness.

**mesothelioma**  A malignant tumor that comes from the mesothelial or lining cells of the pleura, peritoneum, or pericardium.

**messenger RNA**  *See* mRNA.

**metastasis**  The movement of bacteria or cancer cells from one part of the body to another.

**methotrexate**  An anticancer and immunosuppressive drug that blocks dihydrofolate reductase and therefore inhibits folic acid metabolism and DNA synthesis.

**microarray**  An analytic system that permits measurement of the relative presence and expression of thousands of genes simultaneously.

**mixed-lineage leukemia (MLL)** A virulent leukemia observed almost exclusively in children under the age of two and usually in infancy.

**MLL** A gene that is invariably the site of chromosome translocation responsible for mixed-lineage leukemia. The translocation occurs in fetal life.

**MLL translocation** The alteration of one MLL gene by fusion to another gene in the process of chromosomal translocation.

**modified radical mastectomy** This procedure includes removal of the entire breast, nipple, and areola and varying amounts of lymph nodes in the underarm region. Muscle is not removed.

**molecular cytogenetics** A means of increasing the speed, sensitivity, and specificity of conventional cytogenetics using fluorescence-tagged gene (DNA) sequences that are hybridized to chromosome preparations made from patient cells.

**monoclonal antibody** An antibody specific to a certain antigen that is created in the laboratory from hybridoma cells, living factories that are formed by the fusion of the spleen cell derived from a mouse immunized with an antigen and a myeloma cell that replicates and produces the antibody continuously.

**MOPP** Mechlorethamine, vincristine (Oncovin), procarbazine, and prednisone; a combination chemotherapeutic treatment for Hodgkin's disease.

**MRI** *See* magnetic resonance imaging.

**mRNA** Messenger RNA, a type of RNA that carries information from DNA to the protein-forming system of the cell.

**multiple endocrine neoplasia (MEN)** A familial syndrome caused by an inherited and acquired loss of MEN1 tumor suppressor genes. The result is benign and malignant tumors of many endocrine glands.

**multiple myeloma** A disease characterized by the infiltration of bone marrow by cancerous plasma cells.

**mutagen** Any agent that causes genetic mutations. Many medicines, chemicals, and physical means such as ionizing radiations and ultraviolet light have this ability.

**mutation** A spontaneous or induced change in the DNA sequence of a gene in an individual organism. Most mutations are harmless, but others lead to serious disease or disability. Such mutations are either inactivating (e.g., destroying the normal function of a gene) or activating (e.g., enhancing the function of a gene). Mutations in germ cells (ova or sperm) cause inherited genetic abnormalities.

**myc** A growth-regulating gene in a class called transcription factors that produces a protein that collaborates in the cell nucleus with other proteins to induce the expression of many genes. Myc is a proto-oncogene. When mutated to a more active form or overexpressed, it becomes an oncogene. High levels of myc protein are seen in several tumors.

**myeloblast** An immature bone marrow cell in the granulocyte series.

**myeloid/lymphoid leukemia (MLL)** Also known as mixed-lineage leukemia.

**myeloma** A tumor of plasma cells originating in cells of the hematopoietic portion of bone marrow.

**Navelbine** A vincristine-like anticancer drug that inhibits cell division. Generic name: vinorelbine.

**neuroblastoma** A malignant tumor composed principally of cells resembling neuroblasts that give rise to cells of the sympathetic nervous system.

**nilotinib** An anticancer drug that inhibits the abl and kit oncoproteins and is potent against chronic myelogenous leukemia and GIST cells. Chemical name: AMN107.

**nitrogen mustard** The first anticancer drug discovered after the use of mustard gas in World War I. Its use is now limited almost entirely to MOPP chemotherapy.

**N-myc** The neuroblastoma-derived form of myc transcription factor gene that acts as an oncogene in human tumors. Also known as myc-N.

**node** A small, rounded structure; a protuberance or swelling.

**nodule** A small cluster of cells.

**nuclear grade** An evaluation of the size and shape of the nucleus in a tumor cell and the percentage of tumor cells that are dividing. Low nuclear grades indicate a cancer that will spread more slowly than those with high nuclear grades.

**Nutlin** An experimental anticancer drug. *See also* mdm2.

**onco** A combining form defined as tumor, swelling, or mass.

**oncogene** A gene that has the ability to induce tumor formation and malignancy. Proteins produced by these genes have tumor-promoting activity.

**oncoprotein** A protein that is coded by an oncogene that may induce new and abnormal tissue formation such as a tumor.

**Oncovin** Vincristine; particularly used in the treatment of ALL and Hodgkin's disease.

**p53** A protein produced by a tumor suppressor gene that induces the death pathway in cells with injured DNA. When absent, cells are less likely to die and therefore become cancerous.

**palpation** Manual examination of the external surface of the body to detect evidence of disease or abnormalities in the internal organs.

**pancreatitis** Inflammation of the pancreas.

**pancytopenia** A reduction in all cellular elements of the blood.

**papilloma virus** Any of a group of viruses that cause papillomas, warts, and cervical cancer in humans and animals.

**parasite** An organism that lives within, upon, or at the expense of another organism and causes harm.

**pathogenesis** The origin and development of a disease.

**PDGFR** *See* platelet-derived growth factor receptor.

**penicillin** One of a group of antibiotics that kills some bacteria and spirochetes. Penicillin is particularly nontoxic for mammalian cells.

**peristalsis** A progressive wavelike movement that occurs involuntarily in hollow tubes of the body, especially the alimentary canal. The movement consists of contraction of the circular muscle above the distention with relaxation of the region immediately distal to the distended portion. The wave causes the contents of the tube to be forced onward. Cajal cells generate peristalsis.

**peritoneum** The membrane lining the abdominal cavity and reflected over the viscera.

**peritonitis** Inflammation of the membrane that lines the abdominal cavity and its viscera.

**PET scan** *See* positron emission tomography.

**phagocyte** A white blood cell that can ingest and destroy microorganisms, damaged cells, and foreign particles.

**pharmacogenetics** The study of hereditary factors that influence the response of individual organisms to drugs.

**Philadelphia chromosome** An abnormally short chromosome 22 in which there is a reciprocal translocation of the distal portion of its long arm to the long arm of chromosome 9 in exchange for the abl gene. It is found in leukocyte cultures of many patients with chronic myelogenous leukemia. The Philadelphia chromosome was the first chromosomal change found to be characteristic of a human cancer.

**plasma** The pale yellow fluid of the blood in which the particulate components are suspended.

**platelet** A round or oval disk found in the blood of vertebrates. Platelets are fragments of megakaryocytes, large cells found in the bone marrow, and they initiate the clotting process.

**platelet-derived growth factor receptor (PDGFR)** A receptor tyrosine kinase overexpressed or subject to activating mutation in a subset of solid tumors including GIST.

**pneumococci** *See Streptococcus pneumoniae.*

**point mutation** A mutation in DNA that involves a single nucleotide and may consist of loss of a nucleotide, substitution of one nucleotide for another, or the insertion of an additional nucleotide.

**polymer** A natural or synthetic substance formed by a combination of two or more molecules of the same substance.

**polyp** A swelling or tumor emanating from a mucous membrane; commonly found in vascular organs such as the nose, uterus, colon, and rectum.

**portacath** A small plastic port to which a catheter is attached and inserted in a vein. The device is placed in the upper chest wall to enable easy administration of intravenous chemotherapy.

**positron emission tomography (PET scan)** A sectional view of the body using glucose labeled with positron-emitting radionuclides. Since cancer cells use glucose more avidly than most normal cells, PET is used to identify and localize tumors and determine their response to treatment.

**PR** Progesterone receptor.

**prednisone** A glucocorticosteroid with the same effects as cortisone.

**procarbazine hydrochloride** An anticancer drug used in treating Hodgkin's disease.

**progesterone** A steroid hormone responsible for changes in the endometrium (the lining cells of the uterus); used to treat patients with menstrual disorders and to manage endometrial carcinoma. In combination with estrogen, it is used for contraception and postmenopausal hormone replacement therapy.

**progesterone receptor positive** The presence or absence of a receptor to the steroid hormone progesterone in breast cancer cells. Tumors with receptors to estrogen, to progesterone, or to both are more responsive to hormone-blocking agents such as tamoxifen than are tumors that lack these receptors.

**promoter** A region of a gene to which transcription factors (proteins) attach and induce expression of the gene into messenger RNA and then to protein.

**prophylactic chemotherapy** The administration of drug therapy in an attempt to prevent the development of further cancer after surgical removal of the primary or to prevent the onset of cancer in patients with very high risk of developing the disease.

**prostate-specific antigen (PSA)** A protein released by prostate cells and detectable in the blood. It is secreted by both benign prostate cells and malignant tumors, but cancerous prostate cells secrete it at much higher levels. Used as a screening test for cancer.

**protean** Capable of changing form; multifaceted.

**protein** One of a large class of complex nitrogenous compounds that are synthesized by all living organisms and yield amino acids when hydrolyzed. Proteins are the products of genes, carry out critical metabolic reactions, induce movement, and regulate thought. They make us what we are.

**proteosome** An enzyme that degrades misfolded or damaged proteins and modulates the quantity of regulatory proteins in the cell. The breakdown of proteins by proteosomes is triggered when damaged proteins are tagged by a marker protein called ubiquitin.

**proto-oncogene** A gene that regulates the growth of cells or the signals that cells send to each other. Mutations in a proto-oncogene convert the proto-oncogene into an oncogene that may cause excessive growth of cells or tissues in several diseases, particularly cancers.

**PSA** *See* prostate-specific antigen.

**pteropterin** The chemical name for folic acid.

**radiation therapy** The use of energy from X-ray or the radioactive decay of atomic nuclei to destroy diseased tissues such as cancers.

**radioactive** Capable of spontaneous emission of alpha, beta, or gamma rays as a result of the disintegration of the nucleus of an atom.

**raf** A member of the ras signaling pathway that regulates cell proliferation and survival.

**ras** *See* H-ras.

**receptor** In cell biology, a structure in the cell membrane or within a cell that combines with a drug, hormone, protein, or infectious agent to alter an aspect of the functioning of the cell.

**reciprocal translocation** Occurs when a segment of one chromosome is exchanged with a segment of another chromosome of a different pair.

**retroviruses** A large group of RNA viruses that are responsible for a wide range of diseases, including AIDS, malignant tumors, and leukemia.

**reverse transcriptase** An enzyme of retroviruses that catalyzes the synthesis of DNA from the RNA of the virus; the reverse of normal transcription.

**rheumatoid arthritis** A chronic disease marked by inflammation of multiple synovial joints.

**RNA** Ribonucleic acid; a nucleic acid found in all living cells. RNA is involved in all stages of protein synthesis as well as in many regulatory and catalytic roles. It consists of adenine, guanine, cytosine, uracil, ribose, and phosphoric acid.

**Rous sarcoma virus (RSV)** A retrovirus; the first demonstration of an oncogenic virus described in 1911 by Peyton Rous.

**RSV** *See* Rous sarcoma virus.

**SAGE** *See* serial analysis of gene expression.

**sarcoma** A cancer arising from mesenchymal tissue such as muscle, bone, or nerve. It may affect the bones, muscles, bladder, kidneys, liver, brain, gastrointestinal tract, lungs, parotids, and spleen.

**sentinel lymph node biopsy** A technique for identifying the initial site of cancer metastasis. After injection of a radioactive tracer or a dye directly into the tumor mass, the tissue is massaged to encourage tracer uptake by lymphatic vessels. The regional nodes are examined and labeled nodes are removed for microscopic examination.

**sentinel node** A lymph node that receives drainage from a tumor and is likely to harbor metastatic disease before cancer cells have the opportunity to spread elsewhere.

**sepsis** A systemic inflammatory response to infection, in which there is fever or hypothermia, low blood pressure, and inadequate blood flow to internal organs. The syndrome is a common cause of death in critically ill patients.

**sequence** The arrangement of components of large molecules such as nucleotides (DNA) and proteins.

**serial analysis of gene expression (SAGE)** A tool that allows the analysis of absolute rather than relative gene expression patterns in cell populations.

**signaling molecules** A chemical released by cells and tissues to stimulate metabolic activities within those tissues or in other parts of the body. Neurotransmitters, hormones, peptides, cytokines, arachidonic acid derivatives, and other chemicals are all signaling molecules.

**signal transduction inhibitor 571 (STI-571)** *See* imatinib.

**single-nucleotide polymorphism (SNP)** DNA sequence variations that occur when a single nucleotide (A, T, C, or G) in the genome sequence is altered. For a variation to be considered an SNP, it must occur in at least 1 percent of the population. The vast majority of SNPs are without clinical consequence, but they may mark a region of a chromosome that may carry a gene that either causes or ameliorates disease.

**smart drug** An anticancer drug that can target the mutant molecules that induce cancer and do no harm to their healthy counterparts.

**sniffing proteins** A colloquialism that describes proteins like p53 that detect DNA mutations and send cells bearing them down the death pathway.

**SNP** *See* single-nucleotide polymorphism.

**sorafenib** Also known as Bay 43-9006; an anticancer drug constructed to inhibit raf, a member of the ras growth-signaling pathway. It is especially designed to treat malignant melanoma and certain kidney cancers.

**src** The first transforming oncogene discovered. It is a mutant tyrosine kinase responsible for the Rous sarcoma in chickens.

**stage 0 breast cancer** Noninvasive breast cancer. Cancer cells show no evidence of breaking out of the duct or invading the normal tissue surrounding the part of the breast where the cancer began. DCIS (ductal carcinoma in situ) is an example of stage 0.

**stage 1 breast cancer** Invasive breast cancer. Cancer cells are breaking through the duct wall or invading the normal tissue surrounding the breast duct. Tumors in stage 1 measure up to 2 centimeters. There is no lymph node involvement.

**stage 2 breast cancer** Invasive breast cancer in which the tumor measures at least 2 centimeters but not more than 5 centimeters or has spread to the lymph nodes under the arm on the same side as the breast cancer.

**stage 3A breast cancer**  Invasive breast cancer in which the tumor measures larger than 5 centimeters or there is significant involvement of lymph nodes. The nodes clump together or stick to one another or the surrounding tissue.

**stage 3B breast cancer**  Invasive breast cancer in which a tumor of any size has spread to the breast skin, chest wall, or internal mammary lymph nodes.

**stage 4 breast cancer**  Invasive breast cancer in which a tumor has spread beyond the breast, underarm, and internal mammary lymph nodes.

**staphylococcus**  Bacteria that appear round and form grapelike clusters that can be viewed under a microscope.

***Staphylococcus aureus***  Often part of resident flora of the skin and the nasal and oral cavities, these bacteria may cause suppurative conditions such as boils and abscesses, as well as hospital-acquired infections, foreign-body infections, and life-threatening pneumonia or sepsis.

**stem cell**  A rare cell in (for example) the bone marrow whose descendents multiply and specialize into all the mature cells found in the blood, including red cells, granulocytes, monocytes, platelets, and lymphocytes. Stem cells can be harvested from bone marrow, embryonic tissues, peripheral blood, or umbilical cord blood and used in hematological transplants. Stem cells are also responsible for cell renewal of most tissues and organs.

**steroid**  Any one of a large group of substances chemically related to sterols, including cholesterol, D vitamins, certain hormones such as cortisone and androgens, and certain carcinogenic substances.

**STI-571 (Gleevec)**  *See* imatinib.

***Streptococcus pneumoniae***  Often part of the transient flora of the upper respiratory tract, it is the causative agent of many types of pneumonia and is associated with other infectious diseases such as septicemia.

**SU11248**  *See* sunitinib.

**sunitinib**  A kit and abl tyrosine kinase inhibitor and anticancer drug for patients with gastrointestinal stromal tumors (GISTs) and chronic myelogenous leukemia. Trade name: Sutent.

**synthesis**  In this context, the development of a molecule from its component parts.

**tamoxifen**  An antiestrogenic anticancer drug that blocks the interaction of estrogen with its receptor. Used to treat and prevent breast cancer.

**Tarceva**  An anticancer drug that inhibits the action of a mutant receptor tyrosine kinase called the epidermal growth factor receptor (EGFR). The mutant receptor is found on the surface of a fraction of lung cancers. Generic name: erlotinib. *See also* Iressa.

**taxane**  An anticancer class of drugs derived from the bark of the yew tree, *Taxus breviflora*. Examples include paclitaxel and docetaxel. Taxanes inhibit the process of cell division. They are used to treat breast, ovarian, and other types of cancer. Trade name: Taxol.

**Taxol**  *See* taxane.

**T-cell**  A lymphoid cell from the bone marrow that migrates to the thymus gland, where it develops into a mature differentiated T-lymphocyte that circulates between blood and lymph, serving as one of the primary cells of the immune response. Mature T-cells are antigen specific; T-cell receptor proteins detect only one antigen.

**TCR**  T-cell receptor.

**tel**  A gene that transcribes a protein that normally down-regulates gene transcription. When tel is damaged by chromosomal translocation in a bone marrow cell, transcription of several genes is increased and leukemia may result.

**testicular leukemia**  Leukemic cells that may invade the testicles in ALL.

**thioguanine**  An antimetabolite anticancer drug.

**thymocyte**  An immature T-cell.

**T-lymphocyte**  *See* T-cell.

**toxicity**  The quality or degree of being poisonous.

**TRAM flaps**  Transverse rectus abdominis musculocutaneous reconstruction flaps. The procedure used to restore the appearance of a breast after mastectomy.

**translocation**  The alteration of a chromosome by transfer of a portion of it either to another chromosome or to another portion of the same chromosome. The latter is called shift or intrachange.

**tuberculosis bacillus**  Bacterium that causes tuberculosis in humans, also known as *Mycobacterium tuberculosis*.

**tumor**  An abnormal mass. Growth or proliferation that is independent of neighboring tissues is characteristic of all tumors, whether benign or malignant.

**tumor suppressor gene**  A large class of normal genes that suppress the growth of cells. When a member of this regulatory system is inadequate or fails, cancer may develop. *See* antioncogen.

**Tykerb**  *See* lapatinib.

**tyrosine**  An amino acid found especially in cheese (*tyros* is the Greek word for "cheese"). Tyrosine is present in many proteins. It serves as a precursor of epinephrine, thyroxine, and melanin and as an acceptor for high-energy phosphorus from ATP under the influence of tyrosine kinase. Ascorbic acid and folic acid are essential for its metabolism.

**tyrosine kinase**  Any of a group of several hundred enzymes that influence signaling between or within cells, particularly those signals that relate to cell growth and death, cellular adhesion and movement, and cellular differentiation. Activating mutations in tyrosine kinases are found in some human diseases including chronic myeloid (myelogenous) leukemia and GIST.

**tyrosine kinase inhibitor**  A drug that interferes with tyrosine kinase function and therefore with cell communication and growth and may prevent tumor growth. Tyrosine kinase inhibitors are used to treat cancers that are driven by mutant or overexpressed tyrosine kinases.

**ultrasonography**  The use of ultrasound to produce an image of an organ or tissue. Ultrasonic echoes are recorded as they return from reflecting or refracting tissues of different densities.

**vascular endothelial growth factor (VEGF)**  A substance made by cells that stimulates new blood vessel formation by interacting with its receptor, VEGFR, a tyrosine kinase.

**VEGF**  *See* vascular endothelial growth factor.

**VEGFR**  Vascular endothelial growth factor receptor.

**Velcade** An anticancer drug for the treatment of multiple myeloma. The drug's mode of action is to inhibit the formation of proteosomes, the intracellular bodies that store degraded proteins. Generic name: bortezomib.

**vincristine** A fraction of an extract obtained from the periwinkle plant, *Vinca rosea*, a species of myrtle. It is a cytotoxic agent that directly inhibits cell division and is used in treating certain types of malignant tumors, particularly ALL and Hodgkin's disease.

**virus** A pathogen made of nucleic acid (DNA or RNA) inside a protein shell, which can grow and reproduce only after infecting a host cell. More than four hundred types of viruses that cause a great variety of illness are known. All of them can attach to cell membranes, enter the cytoplasm, take over cellular functions, reproduce their parts, and assemble themselves into mature forms capable of infecting other cells. Some of the most virulent agents known are viruses such as the Ebola virus. However, viruses are also responsible for the common cold, childhood exanthems (chickenpox, measles, rubella), latent infections (herpes simplex), some cancers or lymphomas (Epstein-Barr virus), and diseases of virtually any organ system of the body.

**vitamin B9** Folic acid important for the production and maintenance of new cells.

**vitamin B12** A cobamide; a red crystalline substance that contains cobalt. It is extracted from the liver and is essential for the formation of blood cells. Its deficiency results in pernicious anemia. The terms *vitamin B12* and *cyanocobalamin* are used interchangeably as the generic term for the cobamides active in humans.

**Wilms' tumor** A rapidly developing tumor of the kidney that usually occurs in children. It is the most common renal tumor of childhood.

**Zofran** A drug that is effective in relieving nausea associated with chemotherapy. Generic name: ondansetron.

# Bibliography

Below is an alphabetized list of references that I have used in the preparation of this book. Though the list is largely drawn from medical literature, important newspaper and magazine articles are also included. Precise reference numbers are not employed to avoid the dryness of a textbook. Readers should understand that books must finally be printed and that the publication process, like the gestation of a baby, takes time. The references included here are as of late August 2006. Inevitably there will be important progress made after that date and prior to publication. I apologize to those who made that progress and are not cited.

For cancer facts and the most recent information on the war on cancer, visit http://training.seer.cancer.gov/module_cancer_disease/unit5_war_on_cancer.html.

Alt FW, et al. Selective multiplication of dihydrofolate reductase genes in methotrexate-resistant variants of cultured murine cells. *J Biol Chem* 1978;253:1357–70.
*The first report of gene amplification as a cause of drug resistance.*

———. Synthesis and degradation of folate reductase in sensitive and methotrexate-resistant lines of S-180 cells. *J Biol Chem* 1976;251:3063–74.
*First measurement of the enzyme with an antibody.*

Amundadottir T, et al. A common variant associated with prostate cancer in European and African populations. *Nat Genet* 2006;10:1038.
*A genetic variant is associated with higher risk of prostate cancer in African Americans.*

Armstrong SA, et al. FLT3 mutations in childhood acute lymphoblastic leukemia. *Blood* 2004;103:3544–6.
*Description of Flt3 mutations in childhood leukemia.*

———. MLL-rearranged leukemias: insights from gene expression profiling. *Semin Hematol* 2003;40:268–73.
*A good review of gene expression profiling.*

———. MLL translocations specify a distinct gene expression profile that distinguishes a unique leukemia. *Nat Genet* 2002;30:41–7.
*The first demonstration of the unique gene expression pattern of MLL.*

Aur RJ, et al. Central nervous system therapy and combination chemotherapy of childhood lymphocytic leukemia. *Blood* 1971;37:272–81.
*Treatment of spinal fluid leukemia with external radiation.*

Bakalar N. Second opinion may aid breast cancer treatment. *New York Times*, December 5, 2006, p. D7.
*Report on a study shows that second opinions in specialized cancer centers can be very beneficial.*

Baker EK, et al. Epigenetic changes to the MDR1 locus in response to chemotherapeutic drugs. *Oncogene* 2005;24:8061–75.
*Hope that it might be possible to lower the action of the pump that removes drugs from leukemic cells.*

Balduzzi A, et al. Chemotherapy versus allogeneic transplantation for very high-risk childhood acute lymphoblastic leukaemia in first complete remission: comparison by genetic randomisation in an international prospective study. *Lancet* 2005;366:635–42.
*A comparison between chemotherapy and marrow transplant for infant leukemia.*

Beecher HK. Clinical research. *N Engl J Med* 1966;274:1354–60.
*Beecher's call for more attention to research ethics.*

Begg CB. The mammography controversy. *Oncologist* 2002;7:174–6.
———. et al. Impact of hospital volume on operative mortality for major cancer surgery. *JAMA* 1998;280:1747–51.
*The relationship of volume to outcome is nonlinear.*

Beresford SA, et al. Low-fat dietary pattern and risk of colorectal cancer: the Women's Health Initiative Randomized Controlled Dietary Modification Trial. *JAMA* 2006;295:643–54.
*Fat in the diet does not influence cancer risk.*

Berry DA, et al. Effect of screening and adjuvant therapy on mortality from breast cancer. *N Engl J Med* 2005;353:1784–92.
*Early detection and prompt adjuvant therapy reduces breast cancer mortality.*

Blattman JN, Greenberg PD. Cancer immunotherapy: a treatment for the masses. *Science* 2004;305:200–5.
*A good review on progress in immunotherapy of cancer.*

Bonadonna G, et al. Adjuvant cyclophosphamide, methotrexate, and fluorouracil in node-positive breast cancer: the results of 20 years of follow-up. *N Engl J Med* 1995;332:901–6.
*Follow-up on the 1976 study.*

———. Combination chemotherapy as an adjuvant treatment in operable breast cancer. *N Engl J Med* 1976;294:405–10.
*Combination chemotherapy extends survival in breast cancer when given right after surgery.*

Brade WP, et al. Dose-response relationship in experimental and clinical oncology. *Cancer Treat Rev* 1984;11:279–83.
*High dose of combinations is most effective.*

Buchdunger E, et al. Selective inhibition of the platelet-derived growth factor signal transduction pathway by a protein-tyrosine kinase inhibitor of the 2-phenylaminopyrimidine class. *Proc Nat Acad Sci* 1995;92:2558–62.
*Discovery of the precursor to Gleevec by screening a cell line containing PDGFR monitored with the 4G10 antibody.*

Burns CM, et al. Does emotional support influence survival? Findings from a longitudinal study of patients with advanced cancer. *Support Care Cancer* 2005;13:295–302.
*The answer is yes.*

Byrne BJ, Garst J. Epidermal growth factor receptor inhibitors and their role in non-small-cell lung cancer. *Curr Oncol Rep* 2005;7:241–7.
*Results of Iressa and Tarceva trials in lung cancer.*

Calderon-Margalit R, Paltiel O. Prevention of breast cancer in women who carry BRCA1 or BRCA2 mutations: a critical review of the literature. *Int J Cancer* 2004; 112:357–64.
*What steps can be taken to reduce the risks in BRCA-negative women.*

Callahan D. *Setting Limits: Medical Goals in an Aging Society.* Washington, D.C.: George-town University Press, 1995.
*Controlling cost is a major issue.*

Canellos GP, et al. Cyclical combination chemotherapy for advanced breast carcinoma. *Br Med J* 1974;1:218–20.
*The first evidence that combination chemotherapy might be effective in breast cancer.*

Capdeville R, et al. Glivec (STI571, imatinib), a rationally developed, targeted anti-cancer drug. *Nat Rev Drug Discov* 2002;1:493–502.
*Good review of the development of Gleevec.*

Carpenter R, Miller WR. Role of aromatase inhibitors in breast cancer. *Br J Cancer* 2005;93(Suppl 1):S1–5.
*Importance of the addition of aromatase (estrogen synthesis) inhibition after tamoxifen.*

Chowdhury S, Ellis P. Extended adjuvant endocrine therapy of early breast cancer. *Curr Med Res Opin* 2005;21:1985–95.
*Importance of estrogen receptor and estrogen synthesis inhibition in breast cancer.*

Chu E, Devita V, eds. *Physicians Cancer Chemotherapy Drug Manual.* New York: Jones and Bartlett, 2005.
*Contains recommendations on cancer chemotherapy by experts.*

Ciardiello F. Epidermal growth factor receptor inhibitors in cancer treatment. *Future Oncol* 2005;21:221–34.
*Good review of various EGFR inhibitors.*

Clarke M, et al. Effects of radiotherapy and of differences in the extent of surgery for early breast cancer on local recurrence and 15-year survival: an overview of the randomised trials. *Lancet* 2005;366:2087–106.
*Good evidence for the benefit of radiation therapy in breast cancer.*

Clinical trial of Iressa. *FDA Consum* 2005 Mar–Apr;39(2):4.
*The gloomy view of the FDA concerning Iressa trials.*

Crabtree JS, et al. Of mice and MEN1: insulinomas in a conditional mouse knockout. *Mol Cell Biol* 2003;23:6075–85.
*Showing that MEN1 is a tumor suppressor gene.*

———. A mouse model of multiple endocrine neoplasia, type 1, develops multiple endocrine tumors. *Proc Natl Acad Sci USA* 2001;98:1118–23.
*Shows that restoration of MEN1 gene stops the cancer.*

Crile G, Jr. Treatment of cancer of the breast; past, present and future. *Cleve Clin Q* 1971;38:47–54.
*Strongly opposed the Halsted procedure.*

Daley GQ, et al. Induction of chronic myelogenous leukemia in mice by the P210bcr/abl gene of the Philadelphia chromosome. *Science* 1990;247:824–30.
*Shows that CML is caused by bcr-abl.*

D'Amico AV, et al. Preoperative PSA velocity and the risk of death from prostate cancer after radical prostatectomy. *N Engl J Med* 2004;351:125–35.
*The rate of change of PSA is more important than the absolute value.*

Danial NN, Korsmeyer SJ. Cell death: critical control points. *Cell* 2004;116:205–19.
*A superb review of the cell death pathways.*

Demetri GD, et al. Efficacy and safety of imatinib mesylate in advanced gastrointestinal stromal tumors. *N Engl J Med* 2002;347:472–80.
*Report on a large experience of Gleevec in GIST.*

Doll R, et al. Mortality in relation to smoking: 50 years' observations on male British doctors. *BMJ* 2004;328:1529–33.
*Follow-up on the classic study that demonstrated the damage done by smoking.*

Druker B. Signal transduction inhibition: results from phase I clinical trials in chronic myeloid leukemia. *Semin Hematol* 2001;38:9–14.
*A review of initial experience with Gleevec.*

————. Circumventing resistance to kinase-inhibitor therapy. *N Engl J Med* 2006; 354:2594.
*A good review of newer drugs that may work when Gleevec does not.*

————, et al. Activity of a specific inhibitor of the BCR-ABL tyrosine kinase in the blast crisis of chronic myeloid leukemia and acute lymphoblastic leukemia with the Philadelphia chromosome. *N Engl J Med* 2001;344:1038–42.
*The first paper to demonstrate the value of Gleevec.*

————, et al. Efficacy and safety of a specific inhibitor of the BCR-ABL tyrosine kinase in chronic myeloid leukemia. *N Engl J Med* 2001;344:1031–7.
*Two papers on Gleevec in the same issue of the journal.*

————, et al. Oncogenes, growth factors, and signal transduction. *N Engl J Med* 1989;321:1383–91.
*The only mention of the vital antibody 4G10 used to screen for Gleevec.*

The editors. Looking back on the millennium in medicine. *N Engl J Med* 2000;342:42–9.
*Looking back on progress.*

Effects of radiotherapy and of differences in the extent of surgery for early breast cancer on local recurrence and 15-year survival: an overview of the randomised trials. Early Breast Cancer Trialists' Collaborative Group. *Lancet* 2005;366:2087–106.
*A study showing the benefits of radiation therapy in breast cancer.*

Elion GB, Hitchings GH. Antagonists of nucleic acid derivatives. V. Pteridines. *J Biol Chem* 1951;188:611–21.
*Discovery of 6-mercaptopurine.*

Elshaikh M, et al. Advances in radiation oncology. *Annu Rev Med* 2006;57:19–31.
*Very good review of progress in radiation therapy.*

Esteller M. Epigenetics provides a new generation of oncogenes and tumour-suppressor genes. *Br J Cancer* 2006;94:179–83.
*Review of how epigenetic changes influence cancer.*

Farber S, et al. Clinical studies of actinomycin D with special reference to Wilms' tumor in children. 1960. *J Urol* 2002;168:2560–2.
*Farber's second big hit.*

———. Temporary remissions in acute leukemia of children produced by folic acid antagonist 4-aminopteroyl–glutamic acid (aminopterin). *N Engl J Med* 1948;238:787–93.
*The classic paper that describes the first use of antimetabolite-based cancer chemotherapy.*

Farmer H, et al. Targeting the DNA repair defect in BRCA mutant cells as a therapeutic strategy. *Nature* 2005;434:917–21.
*How exploitation of poor DNA repair can lead to cancer treatment.*

Ferrando AA, et al. Gene expression signatures in MLL-rearranged T-lineage and B-precursor acute leukemias: dominance of HOX dysregulation. *Blood* 2003;102:262–8.
*Some of the gene expression abnormalities in MLL that can be exploited therapeutically.*

Fisher B, et al. Tamoxifen for the prevention of breast cancer: current status of the National Surgical Adjuvant Breast and Bowel Project P-1 study. *J Natl Cancer Inst* 2005;97:1652–62.
*The paper that proved that estrogen blockade improves outcome of many breast cancers.*

Fisher RI. CHOP chemotherapy as standard therapy for treatment of patients with diffuse histiocytic lymphoma. *Important Adv Oncol* 1990;217–25.
*Application of combination chemotherapy in lymphoma.*

Fletcher JA, et al. Translocation (9;22) is associated with extremely poor prognosis in intensively treated children with acute lymphoblastic leukemia. *Blood* 1991;77:435–9.
*Some translocations confer very poor prognosis in leukemia.*

Folkman J. Anti-angiogenesis: new concept for therapy of solid tumors. *Ann Surg* 1972;175:409–16.
*First statement by anyone that tumors might be attacked by shrinking their blood vessels.*

Frei E III, Freireich EJ. The clinical cancer researcher—still an embattled species. *J Clin Oncol* 1993;11:1639–51.
*Describes the opposition to their ideas in the cancer establishment.*

———. Leukemia. *Sci Am* 1964;210:88–96.
*Review of inch-by-inch progress.*

———. Progress and perspectives in the chemotherapy of acute leukemia. *Adv Chemother* 1965;2:269–98.
*Review of inch-by-inch progress.*

———, et al. The effectiveness of combinations of antileukemic agents in inducing and maintaining remission in children with acute leukemia. *Blood* 1965;26:642–56.
*Application of Skipper and Schabel's theories to clinical management.*

Freireich EJ, et al. A comparative study of the effect of transfusion of fresh and preserved whole blood on bleeding in patients with acute leukemia. *N Engl J Med* 1959;260:6–11.
*Early study of transfusion support in childhood leukemia.*

———. A distinctive type of intracerebral hemorrhage associated with "blastic crisis" in patients with leukemia. *Cancer* 1960;13:146–54.
*Initial report of a terrible complication.*

Fries DM, et al. Autologous apoptotic cell engulfment stimulates chemokine secretion by vascular smooth muscle cells. *Am J Pathol* 2005;167:345–53.
*The process of engulfment of dead cells produces a release of proteins involved in inflammation; a reason why chemotherapy is so toxic.*

Frontiers of Cancer Research. *Science* 2006;312:1162–78.
*A good up-to-date review of progress.*

Fujiwara T, et al. Cytokinesis failure generating tetraploids promotes tumorigenesis in p53-null cells. *Nature* 2005;437:1043.
*Shows that cells with a deficient death pathway become cancerous when they cannot cleanly divide their chromosomes.*

Gaynon PS. Childhood acute lymphoblastic leukaemia and relapse. *Br J Haematol* 2005;131:579–87.
*A good review of treatment issues.*

Gerber B, et al. Complementary and alternative therapeutic approaches in patients with early breast cancer: a systematic review. *Breast Cancer Res Treat* 2005;95:1–11.
*The positive effects of complementary therapy and some of the risks.*

Gilliland DG, Griffin JD. Role of FLT3 in leukemia. *Curr Opin Hematol* 2002;9:274–81.
*Review of flt3 in adult leukemia.*

———, et al. The molecular basis of leukemia. *Hematology* (Am Soc Hematol Educ Program) 2004;80–97.
*An excellent review.*

Goldin A. Preclinical chemotherapy: historical aspects. *Mt Sinai J Med* 1985;52:419–25.
*Review of the mouse data that led to combination chemotherapy in humans.*

Gopal AK, et al. High-dose radioimmunotherapy versus conventional high-dose therapy and autologous hematopoietic stem cell transplantation for relapsed follicular non-Hodgkin lymphoma: a multivariable cohort analysis. *Blood* 2003;102:2351–7.
*Use of radioactive monoclonal antibodies.*

Goss PE, et al. Randomized trial of letrozole following tamoxifen as extended adjuvant therapy in receptor-positive breast cancer: updated findings from NCIC CTG MA.17. *J Natl Cancer Inst* 2005;97:1262–71.
*Classic article showing benefit of adding an aromatase (estrogen synthesis) inhibitor after five years of tamoxifen.*

Grady D. Racial component is found in a lethal breast cancer. *New York Times*, June 7, 2006, p 16.
*Gene expression in African American women is associated with aggressive breast cancer.*

Greaves MF. Biological models for leukaemia and lymphoma. *IARC Sci Publ* 2004;157:351–72.
*A superb review by a deep thinker in the leukemia field.*

———. *Cancer: the Evolutionary Legacy.* Oxford, England: Oxford University Press, 2000.
*A very well-written and thoughtful treatise.*

Gunsalus CK, et al. Mission creep in the IRB world. *Science* 2006;312:1441.
*A plea to reduce the scope of IRBs.*

Hahn WC, et al. Creation of human tumour cells with defined genetic elements. *Nature* 1999;400:464–8.
*All three Hahn articles review the work of Hahn and Weinberg on the relatively small complement of genes required to initiate and maintain cancer despite widespread chromosome damage.*

Hahn WC, Weinberg RA. Modelling the molecular circuitry of cancer. *Nat Rev Cancer* 2002;2:331–41.
———. Rules for making human tumor cells. *N Engl J Med* 2002;347:1593–1603.

Haiman CA, et al. Ethnic and racial differences in the smoking-related risk of lung cancer. *N Engl J Med* 2006;354:333–42.
*African Americans and Native Hawaiians are more susceptible to tobacco-induced lung cancer than Caucasians and Japanese.*

Hanahan D, Weinberg RA. The hallmarks of cancer. *Cell* 2000;100:57–70.
*A classic description of cancer as an organ within an organ.*

Harris JR, et al. *Diseases of the Breast*, 2nd ed. New York: Lippincott Williams and Wilkins, 2000.
*A classic textbook on breast cancer.*

Harris SL, Levine AJ. The p53 pathway: positive and negative feedback loops. *Oncogene* 2005;24:2899–908.
*Review of p53 by those who were among the first to report it.*

Henderson IC. Aromatase inhibitors in the management of early breast cancer: optimizing the clinical benefit. *Semin Oncol* 2004;31(6 Suppl 12):31–4.
*A good review of estrogen synthesis inhibition in breast cancer.*

Henschke CI, et al. Survival of patients with stage 1 lung cancer detected on CT scanning. *New Eng J Med* 2006;355:1763–71.
*Initial report on the benefits of yearly CT scanning to prolong survival in patients at risk of lung cancer.*

[No authors listed] Herceptin and early breast cancer: a moment for caution. *Lancet* 2005;366:1673.
*Doubts are expressed that Herceptin is effective as an adjuvant.*

Hicks N. Reparations are asked for men who survived syphilis study. *New York Times*, August 16, 1973, p. 14.
*The infamous Tuskegee experiment.*

Hiddemann W. Cytosine arabinoside in the treatment of acute myeloid leukemia: the role and place of high-dose regimens. *Ann Hematol* 1991;62:119–28.
*High-dose AraC in AML.*

The Hill-Burton Free Care Program. HRSA. U.S. Department of Health and Human Services. May 2003. www.hrsa.gov/osp/dfcr/about/aboutdiv.htm.

Hobson K. Cutting the fat won't cut it. A major new study discounts the protective benefits of a low-fat diet. *US News World Rep* 2006;140:64.

Hodi FS, Dranoff G. Combinatorial cancer immunotherapy. *Adv Immunol* 2006;90:341–68.
*Approaches to cancer immunotherapy.*

Huggins C, Bergenstal DM. Inhibition of human mammary and prostatic cancers by adrenalectomy. *Cancer Res* 1952;12:134–41.
*The early days before effective estrogen blockade with drugs.*

Hu M, et al. Distinct epigenetic changes in the stromal cells of breast cancers. *Nat Genet* 2005;37:899–905.
*More evidence that the environment in which a cancer grows influences its behavior through epigenetic changes in gene expression.*

Huizinga JD, et al. W/kit gene required for interstitial cells of Cajal and for intestinal pacemaker activity. *Nature* 1995;373:347–9.
*Kit is required for Cajal cell function and intestinal motility.*

Huntly BJ, Gilliland DG. Cancer biology: summing up cancer stem cells. *Nature* 2005; 435:1169–70.
*An excellent review of the possible role of stem cells in cancer.*

Joensuu H, et al. Effect of the tyrosine kinase inhibitor STI571 in a patient with a metastatic gastrointestinal stromal tumor. *N Engl J Med* 2001;344:1052–6.
*First report of the effects of Gleevec on GIST.*

Joffe S, et al. Satisfaction of the uncertainty principle in cancer clinical trials: retrospective cohort analysis. *BMJ* 2004;328:1463–6.
*Entrance into clinical trials provides benefit if the trials themselves are successful and improve results.*

Jones PA. Overview of cancer epigenetics. *Semin Hematol* 2005;42:S3–8.
*A good review of a complex topic.*

Jordan VC. Chemoprevention with antiestrogens: the beginning of the end for breast cancer. Daniel G. Miller Lecture. *Ann NY Acad Sci* 2001;952:60–72.
*A somewhat optimistic account.*

Juweid ME, Cheson BD. Positron-emission tomography and assessment of cancer therapy. *N Engl J Med* 2006;354:496–507.
*Good description of the PET scanner.*

Kantarijian H, et al. Nilotinib in imatinib-resistant CML and Philadelphia chromosome-positive ALL. *N Engl J Med* 2006;354:2596–8.
*Another example of overcoming Gleevec resistance with new drugs.*

Kitamura Y, Hirotab S. Kit as a human oncogenic tyrosine kinase. *Cell Mol Life Sci* 2004;61:2924–31.
*Kitamura's detection of the role of kit in GIST.*

Kohl NE, et al. Activated expression of the N-myc gene in human neuroblastomas and related tumors. *Science* 1984;226:1335–7.
*Among the first reports to show that myc amplification causes neuroblastoma.*

———. Transposition and amplification of oncogene-related sequences in human neuroblastomas. *Cell* 1983;35:359–67.
*Another report showing that neuroblastoma is due to myc amplification.*

Kohler G, Milstein C. Continuous cultures of fused cells secreting antibody of prede-
fined specificity. *Nature* 1975;256:495–7.
*The first description of monoclonal antibodies.*

Kolata G. Does stress cause cancer? Probably not. *New York Times*, November 29, 2005,
p D1.
*A careful reporter reviews the literature on stress and cancer and finds it wanting.*

———. Hope in the lab. *New York Times*, May 3, 1998.
*A reporter describes anti-angiogenesis.*

———. Reversing trend, big drop is seen in breast cancer. *New York Times*, December
15, 2006, p. 1.
*Report of a study shows that the incidence of breast cancer has dropped by 7 percent as
women cease taking hormone pills at menopause.*

———. Shift in treating breast cancer is under debate. *New York Times*, May 12,
2006, p 1.
*Good description of an important debate.*

———. Slowly cancer genes tender their secrets. *New York Times*, December 27,
2005, p D1.
*A clear report on gene expression in cancer.*

———. Which of these foods will stop cancer (not so fast). *New York Times*, September
27, 2004, p D1.
*The evidence for any effect of diet on cancer incidence is weak.*

Konecny GE. Activity of the dual kinase inhibitor lapatinib (GW572016) against Her-
2-overexpressing and trastuzumab-treated breast cancer cells. *Cancer Res*
2006;66:1630–9.
*First experience with a small molecule that inhibits Her2/neu.*

Kopans DB. The most recent breast cancer screening controversy about whether mam-
mographic screening benefits women at any age: nonsense and nonscience. *Am J
Roentgenol* 2003;180:21–6.
*A rejection of the statistical analyses that lowered the value of mammography.*

Korsmeyer SJ. Bcl-2 initiates a new category of oncogenes: regulators of cell death.
*Blood* 1992;80:879–86.
*The classic review of Korsmeyer's initial findings.*

Kotzerke J, et al. Radioimmunoconjugates in acute leukemia treatment: the future is
radiant. *Bone Marrow Transplant* 2005;36:1021–6.
*How radioactive antibodies can be used in treatment.*

Kriege M, et al. and the Magnetic Resonance Imaging Screening Study Group. Efficacy
of MRI and mammography for breast-cancer screening in women with a familial
or genetic predisposition. *N Engl J Med* 2004;351:427–37.
*MRI is preferred in this very high-risk setting.*

Krivtsov AV, et al. Transformation from committed progenitorto leukaemia stem cell
initiated by MLL-AF9. *Nature* 2006;442:818–22.
*How the MLL translocation produces a highly resistant leukemia.*

Krop I, et al. Frequent HIN-1 promoter methylation and lack of expression in multiple human tumor types. Mol Cancer Res 2004;2:489–94.
*Shows epigenetic influence on cancer gene expression.*

Labialle S, et al. Gene therapy of the typical multidrug resistance phenotype of cancers: a new hope? *Semin Oncol* 2005;32:583–90.
*Attempts to deal with the pump that removes drugs from cancer cells.*

Lamb J. The Connectivity Map: using gene-expression signatures to connect small molecules, genes, and disease. *Science* 2006;313:1929–35.
*A computerized connection of gene-expression data in human cells to available drugs that might lead to new treatment opportunities.*

Lansky SB, et al. Childhood cancer: parental discord and divorce. *Pediatrics* 1978;62:184–8.
*The destructive effects of childhood cancer on family dynamics.*

Laszlo J. *The Cure of Childhood Leukemia: Into the Age of Miracles*. New Brunswick, NJ: Rutgers University Press, 1995.
*An excellent account of the early days by one who was there.*

Lau SC, et al. Technology evaluation: VEGF Trap (cancer), Regeneron/Sanofi-Aventis. *Curr Opin Mol Ther* 2005;7:493–501.
*Review of an interesting approach that works in mice if not in humans.*

Law LW, Boyle PJ. Development of resistance to folic acid antagonists in a transplantable lymphoid leukemia. *Proc Soc Exp Biol Med* 1950;74:599–602.
*Early description of resistance to single agents.*

Leaf C. Why we're losing the war on cancer (and how to win it). *Fortune*, March 22, 2004, pp 77–96.
*A gloomy view of progress.*

Leder A, et al. Consequences of widespread deregulation of the c-myc gene in transgenic mice: multiple neoplasms and normal development. *Cell* 1986;45:485–95.
*Showing how dysregulation of myc can cause cancer.*

Li A, et al. Distinctive IGH gene segment usage and minimal residual disease detection in infant acute lymphoblastic leukaemias. *Br J Haematol* 2005;131:185–92.
*Use of molecular cytogenetics to establish prognosis.*

Li MC, et al. Therapy of choriocarcinoma and related trophoblastic tumors with folic acid and purine antagonists. *N Engl J Med* 1958;259:66–74.
*The first article to show that methotrexate can treat and even cure a solid tumor.*

Lowenbraun S, et al. Combination chemotherapy with nitrogen mustard, vincristine, procarbazine, and prednisone in lymphosarcoma and reticulum cell sarcoma. *Cancer* 1970;25:1018–25.
*Expanding combination chemotherapy into the lymphomas.*

Lux MP, et al. Hereditary breast and ovarian cancer: review and future perspectives. *J Mol Med* 2006;84:16–28.
*An excellent review.*

Lyall S. Court backs Briton's right to a costly drug. *New York Times*, April 13, 2006, p 1.
*Challenge to cost control in Scotland; refusal to pay for Herceptin.*

Lynch TJ, et al. Activating mutations in the epidermal growth factor receptor underlying responsiveness of non-small-cell lung cancer to gefitinib. *N Engl J Med* 2004;350:2129–39.
*Shows that patients with activating mutations benefit from Iressa.*

Marshall J. The role of bevacizumab as first-line therapy for colon cancer. *Semin Oncol* 2005;32:43–7.
*Avastin may be effective when given with chemotherapy.*

McLean TW, et al. TEL/AML-1 dimerizes and is associated with a favorable outcome in childhood acute lymphoblastic leukemia. *Blood* 1996;88:4252–8.
*The tel gene mutation is associated with an improved prognosis.*

Milazzo S, et al. Efficacy of homeopathic therapy in cancer treatment. *Eur J Cancer* 2005;42:282–9.
*Homeopathic therapy is not effective.*

Mintz U, et al. Evolution of karyotypes in Philadelphia (Ph1) chromosome–negative chronic myelogenous leukemia. *Cancer* 1979;43:411–6.
*As CML advances, the chromosome damage worsens.*

Mouridsen HT, Robert NJ. Benefit with aromatase inhibitors in the adjuvant setting for postmenopausal women with breast cancer. *MedGen* 2005;7:20.

———. The role of aromatase inhibitors as adjuvant therapy for early breast cancer in postmenopausal women. *Eur J Cancer* 2005;41:1678–89.
*Both Mouridsen articles show that aromatase (estrogen synthesis) inhibition is highly effective in breast cancer.*

*Nat Rev Cancer* 2004;4:Issues 1–12.
*Review of new drugs.*

NCI study: more than 2 million U.S. women could benefit from tamoxifen. *FDA Consum* 2003;37:7.
*Results of the trial show that tamoxifen reduces breast cancer risk in high-risk patients.*

*Nobel Lectures, Physiology or Medicine 1963–1970.* Amsterdam: Elsevier Publishing Company, 1972. http://nobelprize.org/nobel_prizes/medicine/laureates/1969/luria-bio.html.
*Biography of Salvatore Luria.*

Nocera J. Learning to live with the cigarette. *New York Times Magazine*, June 18, 2006, p 46.
*The ravages of tobacco.*

Nowell PC, Hungerford DA. Chromosome studies on normal and leukemic human leukocytes. *J Nat Cancer Inst* 1960:25;85–109.
*The initial description of the Philadelphia chromosome.*

*Nurse Practitioner Manual of Clinical Skills.* Philadelphia: WB Saunders, 2001.
*Details the role of nurse clinicians in cancer management.*

Odelberg W, ed. http://nobelprize.org/nobel_prizes/medicine/laureates/1975/dulbecco-autobio.html.
*Autobiography of Renato Dulbecco.*

Paez JG, et al. EGFR mutations in lung cancer: correlation with clinical response to gefitinib therapy. *Science* 2004;304:1497–500.
*Shows that patients with activating mutations benefit from Iressa.*

Pan C, et al. Concordance among gene expression based predictors for breast cancer. *N Engl J Med* 2006;355:615–18.
*Several groups confirm each other's results.*

Panel Urges Approval of Vaccine for Cancer. *New York Times*, May 19, 2006.
*Finally, the FDA begins to relent and drop opposition to vaccination to prevent cervical cancer.*

Panka DJ, et al. The Raf inhibitor BAY 43-9006 (sorafenib) induces caspase-independent apoptosis in melanoma cells. *Cancer Res* 2006;66:1611–9.
*Inhibition of raf can cause certain cancer cells to die.*

Paoletti R, et al. *Women's Health and Menopause: Risk Reduction Strategies—Improved Quality of Health.* Norwell, MA: Kluwer Academic Publishers, 1999.

Parada LF, et al. Human EJ bladder carcinoma oncogene is homologue of Harvey sarcoma virus ras gene. *Nature* 1982;297:474–8.
*The point mutation that causes human bladder cancer.*

Pearson HA. History of pediatric hematology oncology. *Pediatr Res* 2002;52:979–92.
*An excellent account of the Sidney Farber period.*

Peppercorn JM, et al. Comparison of outcomes in cancer patients treated within and outside clinical trials: conceptual framework and structured review. *Lancet* 2004;363:263–70.
*Better clinical results are not always seen in patients who are enrolled in clinical trials.*

Piccart-Gebhart MJ, et al. Herceptin Adjuvant (HERA) Trial Study Team. Trastuzumab after adjuvant chemotherapy in Her2-positive breast cancer. *N Engl J Med* 2005; 353:1659–72.
*Confirms article by Romond et al.*

———. Trastuzumab after adjuvant chemotherapy in Her2-positive breast cancer. *N Engl J Med* 2005;353:1659–72.
*The promise of Herceptin as adjuvant therapy for Her/2 neu-positive breast cancer.*

Pieters R, et al. Relation between age, immunophenotype and in vitro drug resistance in 395 children with acute lymphoblastic leukemia—implications for treatment of infants. *Leukemia* 1998;12:1344–8.
*The Dutch experience with MLL therapy.*

Pohlman B, et al. Review of clinical radioimmunotherapy. *Expert Rev Anticancer Ther* 2006;6:445–61.
*How radioactive antibodies kill cancer cells.*

Pollack A. FDA restricts access to cancer drug, citing ineffectiveness. *New York Times*, June 18, 2005.
*Threat to continued use of Iressa.*

———. New drug holds promise for type of breast cancer. *New York Times*, June 4, 2006, p 20.
*The promise of Herceptin as adjuvant therapy for Her/2 neu-positive breast cancer.*

————. New drugs for cancer could soon flood the market. *New York Times*, June 5, 2006, p C1.
*Enthusiastic report on progress.*

Polyak K. On the birth of breast cancer. *Biochim Biophys Acta* 2001;1552:1–13.
*A review of Polyak's early work.*

————, Riggins GJ. Gene discovery using the serial analysis of gene expression technique: implications for cancer research. *J Clin Oncol* 2001;19:2948–58.
*Finding cancer genes with SAGE.*

Popescu NC, Zimonjic DB. Chromosome-mediated alterations of the myc gene in human cancer. *J Cell Mol Med* 2002;6:151–9.
*Chromosome rearrangements, viral integrations, or epigenetic changes can induce high myc expression and cancer.*

Porter D, et al. A neural survival factor is a candidate oncogene in breast cancer. *Proc Natl Acad Sci USA* 2003;100:10931–6.
*Finding a cancer gene that causes DCIS cells to become more malignant.*

Potti A, et al. A genomic strategy to refine prognosis in early-stage non-small cell lung cancer. *N Engl J Med* 2006;355:618–24.
*Gene expression profiles predict survival in lung cancer.*

Prentice RL, et al. Low-fat dietary pattern and risk of invasive breast cancer: the Women's Health Initiative Randomized Controlled Dietary Modification Trial. *JAMA* 2006;295:629–42.
*No influence of low-fat diet on cancer.*

Pui CH, et al. Acute lymphoblastic leukemia. *N Engl J Med* 2004;350:1535–48.
*A very good review of ALL.*

Quackenbush J. Microarray analysis and tumor classification. *N Engl J Med* 2006;354: 2463–72.
*A careful review of the mathematics involved in measurements of gene expression.*

Queller, J. Cancer and the maiden. *New York Times*, March 5, 2005.
*The saga of a woman with inherited susceptibility to breast and ovarian cancer.*

Radeva JI, et al. National estimates of the use of hematopoietic stem-cell transplantation in children with cancer in the United States. *Bone Marrow Transplant* 2005;36: 397–404.
*How bone marrow transplant is used in childhood leukemia.*

Raloff J. Sun struck: data suggest skin cancer epidemic looms. *Science News* online, August 13, 2005.
*A way to prevent cancer.*

Reddy GK, Bukowski RM. Sorafenib: recent update on activity as a single agent and in combination with interferon-alpha2 in patients with advanced-stage renal cell carcinoma. *Clin Genitourin Cancer* 2006;4:246–8.
*More work on combinations of VEGFR inhibition and a general cell suppressor.*

Richardson PG, et al. New treatments for multiple myeloma. *Oncology* 2005;19:1781–92.
*A good review of new approaches to the treatment of multiple myeloma.*

Richmond JB, Fein R. *The Health Care Mess*. Cambridge, MA: Harvard University Press, 2005.
*A very discouraging look at health care.*

Rieselbach RE, et al. Intrathecal aminopterin therapy of meningeal leukemia. *Arch Intern Med* 1963;111:620–30.
*Treatment of spinal fluid leukemia with methotrexate.*

Romond EH, et al. Trastuzumab plus adjuvant chemotherapy for operable Her2-positive breast cancer. *N Engl J Med* 2005;353:1673–84.
*Herceptin given at surgery definitely prolongs survival in Her2/neu-positive breast cancer.*

Rous P. A transmissible avian neoplasm. (Sarcoma of the common fowl) by Peyton Rous, M.D., *Experimental Medicine* for September 1, 1910, vol. 12, pp 696–705. *J Exp Med* 1979;150:738–53.
*Description of Rous's early work.*

Sanborn RE, Sandler AB. The safety of bevacizumab. *Expert Opin Drug Safety* 2006;5:289–301.
*The safety of anticancer treatment with a monoclonal antibody.*

Sansam CG, Roberts CW. Epigenetics and cancer: altered chromatin remodeling via Snf5 loss leads to aberrant cell cycle regulation. *Cell Cycle* 2006;5:621–4.
*The complex role of epigenetics in cancer.*

Schabel FM Jr, et al. Concepts for controlling drug-resistant tumor cells. *Eur J Cancer* 1980(Suppl 1):199–211.
*The voice of the other partner in the Skipper-Schabel alliance at Southern Research Institute.*

Schimke RT, et al. Studies on the amplification of dihydrofolate reductase genes in methotrexate-resistant cultured mouse cells. *Cold Spring Harb Symp Quant Biol* 1979;43(Pt 2):1297–303.
*The work that stimulated Fred Alt to move forward to define the cause of methotrexate resistance.*

Schoffski P, et al. Emerging role of tyrosine kinase inhibitors in the treatment of advanced renal cell cancer: a review. *Ann Oncol* January 17, 2006 [Epub ahead of print].
*A review of the progress in producing tyrosine kinase inhibitors in cancer.*

Sengupta S, et al. Temporal targeting of tumour cells and neovasculature with a nanoscale delivery system. *Nature* 2005;436:568–72.
*A novel drug combination.*

Shaughnessy D. Jimmy Fund gets 50th anniversary gift: "Jimmy." *Boston Globe*, May 17, 1998.
*Return of Eynar Gustaffson (Jimmy) to Fenway Park.*

Shih C, et al. Passage of phenotypes of chemically transformed cells via transfection of DNA and chromatin. *Proc Natl Acad Sci USA* 1979;76:5714–18.
*DNA of cancer cells transferred into normal cells turns the normal cells into cancer cells.*

A short history of the National Institutes of Health. Office of NIH History, http://history.nih.gov/exhibits/history/.
*A useful review of the history of the National Institutes of Health.*

Siegal-Lakhai WS, et al. Current knowledge and future directions of the selective epidermal growth factor receptor inhibitors erlotinib (Tarceva) and gefitinib (Iressa). *Oncologist* 2005;10:579–89.
*How these drugs work in lung cancer.*

Siegel B. *Peace, Love and Healing.* New York: HarperCollins, 1989.
*A well-known physician speaks of easing pain and suffering in cancer patients.*

Silverman LB, et al. Clinical observations, interventions, and therapeutic trials. Improved outcome for children with acute lymphoblastic leukemia: results of Dana-Farber Consortium Protocol 91-01. *Blood* 2001;97:1211–18.
*Reviews improving results.*

———. Intensified therapy for infants with acute lymphoblastic leukemia: results from the Dana-Farber Cancer Institute Consortium. *Cancer* 1997;80:2285–95.
*How intensification improved survival in high-risk patients.*

Singer S, et al. Prognostic value of KIT mutation type, mitotic activity, and histologic subtype in gastrointestinal stromal tumors. *J Clin Oncol* 2002;20:3898–905.
*The relationship of kit mutation to the severity of GIST.*

Sinn E, et al. Coexpression of MMTV/v-Ha-ras and MMTV/c-myc genes in transgenic mice: synergistic action of oncogenes in vivo. *Cell* 1987;49:465–75.
*Showing that more than one abnormal gene may be required to unleash cancer.*

Skipper HE. Experimental adjuvant chemotherapy: an overview. *Recent Results Cancer Res* 1986;103:6–29.
*A review of Skipper and Schabel's work that supported the use of combination chemotherapy.*

———. Laboratory models: some historical perspective. *Cancer Treat Rep* 1986;70:3–7.
*How animal models show the way to improved treatment.*

Slamon DJ. The future of ErbB-1 and ErbB-2 pathway inhibition in breast cancer: targeting multiple receptors. *Oncologist* 2004;9:1–3.
*Review by the investigator who first brought Herceptin forward into therapy.*

Solovyan VT, Keski-Oja J. Apoptosis of human endothelial cells is accompanied by proteolytic processing of latent TGF-beta binding proteins and activation of TGF-beta. *Cell Death Differ* 2005;12:815–26.
*More evidence that the process of engulfment of dead cells releases toxic proteins.*

Spicer J, et al. Adjuvant trastuzumab for Her2-positive breast cancer. *Lancet* 2005;366:634.
*Casting doubt.*

Stam RW, et al. Differential mRNA expression of Ara-C-metabolizing enzymes explains Ara-C sensitivity in MLL gene-rearranged infant acute lymphoblastic leukemia. *Blood* 2003;101:1270–6.
*AraC is actually pumped into MLL cells.*

———. Targeting Flt3 in primary MLL-gene-rearranged infant acute lymphoblastic leukemia. *Blood* 2005;106:2484–90.
*Shows that Flt3 mutant MLL leukemia cells can be readily killed with a smart drug.*

Stephens P, et al. A screen of the complete protein kinase gene family identifies diverse patterns of somatic mutations in human breast cancer. *Nature Genetics* 2005;37:590–2.

*The known protein kinase genes of sixteen primary invasive ductal breast cancers were sequenced by the Sanger Laboratory. No mutations were found in twelve of the tumors. Two had a single mutation and one had two mutations. A single case had fifty-two mutations. The observed mutations were highly variable from one cancer to another. This preliminary study suggests that there is no commonly point-mutated and activated protein kinase gene in invasive ductal breast cancer. Amplification of the Her2/neu gene is by far the most important kinase defect to cause breast cancer.*

Stewart T, et al. Spontaneous mammary adenocarcinomas in transgenic mice that carry and express MTV/myc fusion genes. *Cell* 1984;38:627–38.
*The first demonstration that high myc expression could cause cancer in an experimental animal.*

Stone RM, et al. Patients with acute myeloid leukemia and an activating mutation in FLT3 respond to a small-molecule FLT3 tyrosine kinase inhibitor, PKC412. *Blood* 2005;105:54–60.
*Flt3 inhibitors have a limited positive effect in AML; resistance is a problem.*

Strickland S. *The History of Regional Medical Programs*. Lanham, MD: University Press of America, 2000.
*A great idea faded away.*

Surowiecki J. Up in smoke. *New Yorker*, November 21, 2005, p 46.
*The politics of tobacco.*

Swanstrom R, et al. Transduction of a cellular oncogene: the genesis of Rous sarcoma virus. *Proc Natl Acad Sci USA* 1983;80:2519–23.
*A study that shows how the normal nononcogenic rous virus can be altered to gain an oncogene when it invades a chicken cell.*

Talpaz M, et. al. Dasatinib in imatinib-resistant Philadelphia chromosome–positive leukemias. *N Engl J Med* 2006;354:2594–6.
*Shows that new drugs can overcome Gleevec resistance.*

Temin HM. Malignant transformation of cells by viruses. *Perspect Biol Med* 1970;14: 11–26.
*Early discussion of reverse transcriptase.*

———. On the origin of the genes for neoplasia: G. H. A. Clowes memorial lecture. *Cancer Res* 1974;34:2835–41.
*A review of Clowes's theory and discovery of reverse transcriptase.*

Toh BH, et al. Pernicious anemia. *N Engl J Med* 1997;337:1441–8.
*A modern review of the field.*

Twombly R. Negative Women's Health Initiative findings stir consternation, debate among researchers. *J Natl Cancer Inst* 2006;98:508–10.
*Diet does not influence cancer incidence.*

van de Vijver MJ, et al. A gene-expression signature as a predictor of survival in breast cancer. *N Engl J Med* 2002;347:1999–2009.
*Shows influence of gene expression on survival.*

van't Veer LJ, et al. Gene expression profiling predicts clinical outcome of breast cancer. *Nature* 2002;415:530–6.

*Gene expression array analysis of breast cancer cells selects the patients with poor prognosis.*

Varley JM. Germline p53 mutations and Li-Fraumeni syndrome. *Hum Mutat* 2003;21:313–20.
*An excellent review of Li-Fraumeni syndrome.*

Varmus H, Weinberg R. *Genes and the Biology of Cancer*. New York: Scientific American Library, 1992.
*A delightful, small, and well-illustrated book on cancer genetics.*

Vassilev LT, et al. In vivo activation of the p53 pathway by small-molecule antagonists of mdm2. *Science* 2004;303:844–8.
*An inhibitor of the protein that binds p53, allows p53 to rise in cancer cells, and thereby kills the tumor.*

Venturini M, et al. Dose-dense adjuvant chemotherapy in early breast cancer patients: results from a randomized trial. *J Natl Cancer Inst* 2005;97:1724–33.
*Decreasing interval of dose has a small benefit.*

Verma IM, et al. Synthesis by reverse transcriptase of DNA complementary to globin messenger RNA. *Basic Life Sci* 1974;3:355–72.
*Use of reverse transcriptase to amplify and label a normal human gene.*

Veronesi U, et al. A randomized comparison of sentinel-node biopsy with routine axillary dissection in breast cancer. *N Engl J Med* 2003;349:546–53.
*An excellent study of the efficacy of sentinel node biopsy.*

Vogelstein B, Kinzler K. Cancer genes and the pathways they control. *Nat Med* 2004;10:789–99.
*A superb review by two well-established experts.*

———. *The Genetic Basis of Human Cancer*, 2nd ed. New York: McGraw-Hill Company, 2002.
*A fine text on cancer.*

Walensky LD, et al. Activation of apoptosis in vivo by a hydrocarbon-stapled BH3 helix. *Science* 2004;305:1466–70.
*A new approach to anticancer drug development.*

*Wall Street Journal*, Editorial, February 23, 2006.
*Enthusiastic report of progress.*

Watson M, et al. Influence of psychological response on breast cancer survival: 10-year follow-up of a population-based cohort. *Eur J Cancer* 2005;41:1710–4.
*Data suggesting that emotions can affect outcome in cancer.*

Wei G, et al. Gene-expression-based chemical genomics identifies rapamycin as a modulator of MCL1 and glucocorticoid resistance. *Cancer Cell* 2006;10:331–42.
*Discovery of a totally unexpected enhancer of corticosteroid therapy in leukemia by use of the Connectivity Map described by Lamb, et al.*

Weinberg R. *The Biology of Cancer*. New York: Garland Science, 2006.
*A classic text.*

Weindling PJ. *Nazi Medicine and the Nurenberg Trials*. New York: Palgrave Macmillan, 2004.
*A sobering review of the conduct of Nazi physicians.*

Welch AD. Folic acid: discovery and the exciting first decade. *Perspect Biol Med* 1983;27:64–75.
*An exciting review of the discovery of folic acid.*

Welch HG. *Should I Be Tested for Cancer?* Berkeley: University of California Press, 2004.
*A challenge to those who believe in screening tests.*

————, et al. Skin biopsy rates and incidence of melanoma: population based ecological study. *BMJ* 2005;331:481.
*No benefit from screening for melanoma.*

Welsh PL, King MC. BRCA1 and BRCA2 and the genetics of breast and ovarian cancer. *Hum Mol Genet* 2001;10:705–13.
*The status of breast and ovarian cancer at the time.*

Wilcox WS, et al. Experimental evaluation of potential anticancer agents. XV. On the relative rates of growth and host kill of "single" leukemia cells that survive in vivo cytoxan therapy. *Cancer Res* 1966;26:1009–14.
*How to get to the last cancer cell.*

Yager JD, Davidson NE. Mechanisms of disease. Estrogen carcinogenesis in breast cancer. *N Engl J Med* 2006;354:270–82.
*A very good review.*

Yano H, et al. Expression and activation of apoptosis-related molecules involved in interferon-alpha-mediated apoptosis in human liver cancer cells. *Int J Oncol* 2005; 26:1645–52.
*The process of engulfment of dead cells produces a release of toxic proteins involved in inflammation.*

Yoshida K, Miki Y. Role of BRCA1 and BRCA2 as regulators of DNA repair, transcription, and cell cycle in response to DNA damage. *Cancer Sci* 2004;95:866–71.
*The two genes are among several that carry out DNA repair. Their absence increases the risk of cancer.*

Young WW, et al. Dissemination of clinical results. Mastectomy versus lumpectomy and radiation therapy. *Med Care* 1996;34:1003–17.
*An important lesson: How long does it take for information to percolate to the practitioner and change his or her behavior?*

# Index